The Diabetes Lifestyle Book

Facing Your Fears &
Making Changes for a
Long & Healthy Life

JENNIFER GREGG, PH.D.
GLENN M. CALLAGHAN, PH.D.
STEVEN C. HAYES, PH.D.

New Harbinger Publications, Inc.

Publisher's Note

Care has been taken to confirm the accuracy of the information presented and to describe generally accepted practices. However, the authors, editors, and publisher are not responsible for errors or omissions or for any consequences from application of the information in this book and make no warranty, express or implied, with respect to the contents of the publication.

The authors, editors, and publisher have exerted every effort to ensure that any drug selection and dosage set forth in this text are in accordance with current recommendations and practice at the time of publication. However, in view of ongoing research, changes in government regulations, and the constant flow of information relating to drug therapy and drug reactions, the reader is urged to check the package insert for each drug for any change in indications and dosage and for added warnings and precautions. This is particularly important when the recommended agent is a new or infrequently employed drug.

Some drugs and medical devices presented in this publication may have Food and Drug Administration (FDA) clearance for limited use in restricted research settings. It is the responsibility of the health care provider to ascertain the FDA status of each drug or device planned for use in their clinical practice.

Acquired by Jess O'Brien; Cover design by Amy Shoup; Edited by Carole Honeychurch; Text design by Tracy Carlson

Library of Congress Cataloging-in-Publication Data

Gregg, Jennifer.
  Diabetes lifestyle book : facing your fears and making changes for a long and healthy life / Jennifer Gregg, Glenn M. Callaghan & Steven C. Hayes.
    p. cm.
  ISBN-13: 978-1-57224-516-7
  ISBN-10: 1-57224-516-6
  1. Diabetes--Treatment--Popular works. 2. Diabetes--Psychological aspects--Popular works. 3. Acceptance and commitment therapy--Popular works. I. Callaghan, Glenn M. II. Hayes, Steven C. III. Title.
  RC660.4.G76 2007
  616.4'6206--dc22

                              2007023351

09 08 07   10 9 8 7 6 5 4 3 2 1   First printing

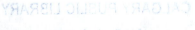

Contents

A Letter from the Series Editors v

Foreword ix

Introduction. 1

PART I
Where We Start

CHAPTER 1
What Is It About Diabetes?. 9

CHAPTER 2
The Basics: Introducing Diabetes. 17

CHAPTER 3
Value Added 37

Part II
Diabetes Acceptance

CHAPTER 4
What Have You Tried? 59

CHAPTER 5
Who Are You? 73

CHAPTER 6
Willing to *What*? 89

Part III
Your Individual Diabetes Plan

CHAPTER 7
Food, Glorious Food 109

CHAPTER 8
Exercise Your Rights 129

CHAPTER 9
Talking Diabetes 145

CHAPTER 10
Medication Meditation 165

CHAPTER 11
Preventing, Detecting, and Treating Complications 181

Part IV
Tying It All Together:
Acceptance + Plan = Commitment

CHAPTER 12
Behavior Change 203

CHAPTER 13
Stand and Commit 215

References 225

Dear Reader:

Welcome to New Harbinger Publications. New Harbinger is dedicated to publishing books based on acceptance and commitment therapy (ACT) and its application to specific areas. New Harbinger has a long-standing reputation as a publisher of quality, well-researched books for general and professional audiences.

This book, *The Diabetes Lifestyle Book*, is an intimately practical and user-friendly guide for those struggling with diabetes and their loved ones. Diabetes, as you may know, is a serious and quite scary medical condition. Nobody asks for it, yet it is there anyway. But it's not a death sentence either. Diabetes is a condition that can be managed, and in many ways must be managed. The complications of unchecked diabetes can do serious damage to you. Those complications can even cut your life short needlessly.

The authors of *The Diabetes Lifestyle Book* draw on the latest research and practical know-how to help you more effectively manage your diabetes (and the barriers that get in the way of that management) with an eye on the prize—helping you live better even with your diabetes. Put another way, this book will help you put diabetes management in its proper context as one part of your life, not the very fabric of who you are.

As you move through the book, you'll learn a number of things. The authors will teach you a bit about diabetes, its complications, and what we know about them. The book, though, is bigger than that. It is about you taking care of yourself so that you can make the most of your one precious life. To get there, the authors will help you take stock of what matters to you—your values.

You'll also have a chance to take a good look at the barriers that seem to be getting in the way of you taking care of your diabetes. If you're like many people with diabetes, we think you'll find that many of the barriers are self-inflicted, products of what your mind and body are telling you—that it's too much, too difficult, too painful, or that nothing will change, so why bother. On top of that, you have legitimate feelings like resentment, guilt, shame, anxiety, sadness, a sense of loss, and even anger. These feelings can leave you feeling hopeless, worn out, and alone.

These barriers are important for one simple reason: they can keep you from taking care of yourself. If you don't attend to them, then you will suffer. And, if you suffer some of the serious medical complications that come along with unchecked diabetes, you won't be able to do what you most care about. In short, when your health suffers needlessly, your life will tend to shrink needlessly. The authors teach us that it doesn't have to be this way. There is a way out.

If you read this book and do the exercises, you stand a great chance of getting your diabetes under control. And, you will learn a powerful set of skills and strategies that will help you keep your health and your life on track in directions you want to go. Here, too, you'll learn how to move with unpleasant barriers rather than having to defeat them in order to create the life that you so desperately want to live. The authors will show you how to have a vital life, even with diabetes, by teaching you how to balance acceptance *and* change. These ideas are not fluff. There is a growing body of research showing that ACT skills and strategies benefit people just like you, as well as those with other serious medical and psychological problems such as multiple sclerosis, cancer, chronic pain, anxiety, depression, and even schizophrenia, one of the more serious and hard-to-treat psychological conditions that we know of.

Why ACT works as well as it does across the gamut of human suffering is being worked out as we speak, but we think it has to do with this: the skills help people get unstuck and moving in ways that are vital, meaningful, and dignified without first having to win the war with unpleasant thoughts, memories, and physical sensations. ACT is not a panacea or cure for your diabetes, but it will help you to put your time and energy into things that you can control and need to control. In short, it will help you live better.

We encourage you to put reading this book on your "take-care-of-yourself to-do list" each day. Work with the material and let it work for you. We know that you didn't ask for diabetes, but we do know this much—you can do something about it. You are much bigger than your diabetes.

We know that some of what you read will be challenging, but the potential payoff is great. We hope that you allow the material in this book to help you take important steps toward a healthier, fuller, and more vital life. Remember that you can take control of your diabetes instead of letting your diabetes control you. This book will show you the way.

As part of New Harbinger's commitment to publishing sound, scientific, clinically based research, Steven C. Hayes, Ph.D., Georg Eifert, Ph.D., and John Forsyth, Ph.D., oversee all prospective ACT books for the Acceptance and Commitment Therapy Series. New Harbinger is at the forefront of publishing books that make ACT skills available to general and professional audiences.

As ACT Series editors, we review all ACT books published by New Harbinger, comment on proposals and offer guidance as needed, and use a gentle hand in making suggestions regarding content, depth, and scope of each book. We strive to ensure that any unsubstantiated claim or claims that are clearly ACT inconsistent are flagged for the authors so they can revise these sections to ensure that the work meets our criteria (see below) and that all of the material presented is true to ACT's roots (not passing off other models and methods as ACT).

Books in the Acceptance and Commitment Therapy Series:

■ Have an adequate database. Those meant for the public will have at least one reasonably well-done and successful randomized trial showing that the methods are helpful.

■ Are theoretically coherent: they will fit with the ACT model and underlying behavioral principles as they have evolved at the time of writing.

■ Refrain from making excessive claims and orient the reader toward unresolved empirical issues.

■ Do not overlap needlessly with existing volumes.

■ Avoid jargon and the needless creation of new terms or unnecessary entanglement with proprietary methods.

- Keep the focus always on what is good for the reader.

- Support the further development of the field.

- Provide information in a way that is of practical use to readers.

These guidelines reflect the values of the broader ACT community. You'll see all of them packed into this book. They are meant to guard against unsubstantiated claims, and to ensure that you get something that can truly be helpful to you. Now, it's time for you to take a look and find out for yourself.

Sincerely,

John Forsyth, Ph.D.
Steven C. Hayes, Ph.D.
Georg H. Eifert, Ph.D.

Foreword

For me, one of the best things about being a physician is helping people in acute situations. A patient shows up at your office, or at the hospital, with severe pain, sudden bleeding, or some other complaint that defies explanation. To an experienced physician, these terrifying symptoms are often familiar, their causes clear, and the solution readily available. Apply your knowledge, review your experience, ply your skills, and you can frequently fix a crisis that was anything from very distressing to nearly fatal.

Before I get too satisfied about deftly putting out a medical fire, I remind myself of a maxim attributed to Anton Chekhov: "Any idiot can face a crisis—it is day-to-day living that wears you out." Chekhov himself was a physician, and his remark recognizes something all health care providers must acknowledge: Acute emergencies make up only a fraction of health care and represent what might be the easiest part of a doctor's job. The rest is chronic, and no chronic condition better reflects this than diabetes mellitus, now largely shorthanded as simply "diabetes."

So if I am the idiot who can handle the crisis, who is the genius to tackle the chronic condition, in this case diabetes? That genius is you, the person with diabetes, or the spouse, the parent, the child, or the friend of the person with diabetes. In receiving a diagnosis of diabetes, you have been granted the opportunity to reveal your genius in managing a complex illness that can affect your whole body. I say "can" rather than "will," because your ability to change your diet, exercise regularly, and keep up with a medication schedule will prevent the deadly complications of diabetes. You have the abilities already; you may just need some help in discovering them.

In this book, Drs. Gregg, Callaghan, and Hayes present the essential tools of diabetes management. By now, you may be familiar with the physiology and complications of this condition; if not, you can learn about them here. What you may not be familiar with—and indeed, your physician probably doesn't know either—are the strategies for coping with your feelings, and with the feelings and assumptions of those close to you, as you take on the challenge of diabetes. Qualified physicians, nurses, educators, and nutritionists can tell you what to eat, how much to walk, and when to drop a glyburide tablet down your throat. They cannot, however, eat for you, move your legs, or pry your gullet open. That's all on you. It's difficult, taken altogether, to do that while living in a society that does little to facilitate your health. But it's not impossible, and you have the equipment. And as this book shows, even what you perceive as the obstacles to accomplishing excellent diabetes self-care—your appetites, your doubts, your regrets, and your anger—can be marshaled to conquer to this condition.

Part of my pleasure in handling a medical emergency is claiming at the end of the day that I saved a life. What all physicians know, though, is that patients save their own lives. Your choices—to quit smoking, to exercise, to eat healthfully, and to work with your doctor—are what keep you alive and make your life worthwhile. Making those choices, and sticking to them, is the hard part. Not impossible, but hard, although much easier than you think, as this book will show. The diagnosis of diabetes can give you the satisfaction of saving a life every day: your own.

—Michael Singer, MD

Introduction

Congratulations. You may have picked this book up because you are a person with diabetes. Or maybe you know or love somebody with diabetes. Or maybe you are, know, or love somebody who is at risk for developing diabetes. Whatever your reason for choosing this book, we congratulate you because picking it up is the first step toward living a vital life with diabetes.

First off, you are not alone. Approximately 20 million people in the United States have diabetes, and another 41 million have "prediabetes"—a condition that often leads to the development of diabetes (Cowie et al. 2006). Finding out you have or are at risk for developing diabetes can be a life-changing experience. For many people this change is viewed in terms of the losses it represents. The loss of chocolate cake or ice cream sundaes, the loss of lazy days lying on the couch, the potential loss of eyesight, limbs, or functioning. The loss of a carefree relationship with food and one's own body. But, as hard as it might be to believe now, the development of diabetes can also represent a gain. Indeed, for some people the development of diabetes is the wake-up call that is needed in order to really begin *living* their life. This represents a transition from a life of existing to a life of living.

Diabetes Is Different

Whatever your relationship with diabetes, one thing we probably don't have to tell you is that diabetes is different from many of the diseases that affect people in our society. What most characterizes this difference is the tremendous amount of self-management required with diabetes. Diabetes is not a disease managed by your doctor on annual or semi-annual clinic visits. It's not a disease where you take a medication until it is gone. It requires large changes in how you eat, exercise, and take care of yourself every day. It can affect what you see, how you get around, how you feel, how you communicate with your spouse, friends, and family, and can even affect your most intimate sexual moments. In essence, every aspect of life changes with this disease, and to manage it requires an enormous amount of dedication, skill, and discipline—commodities in short supply for most of us.

In addition to this enormous management component, another aspect of diabetes that makes it different from other diseases is the fact that it is the *complications* of diabetes, brought about by high or low blood sugar, that cause problems for people rather than the disease itself. This means that many people live with diabetes for decades without suffering the painful effects, as long as good blood sugar control is achieved.

This situation creates a high level of stress. To complicate matters even more, how you react to this stress, as well as the general stress experienced in life, influences your blood sugar. Different mechanisms have been put forth for why this might be the case, but the bottom line is that whether it's because effective coping skills allow you to do a better job of managing the disease, or because coping skills have a direct effect on blood sugar and other body effects, we know that how you cope with the stressors in your life matters in managing blood sugar.

So the situation is this: 1) you have a chronic disease that you have primary responsibility for managing; 2) the management of this disease is very complex; 3) if you do not manage it well, you may develop complications that could be fatal; and 4) although this is a stressful situation, you should not experience too much stress about it, because stress could make things worse.

Coping with Feelings

The enormity of these factors can be too much for many people with diabetes to handle. You may understandably hope for this problem to go away, or that you have been misdiagnosed. You might have difficulty dealing with the reality of the situation because maybe you do not *feel* any different. One of the cruel tricks diabetes plays is that you frequently don't feel any physically different than you did before you were diagnosed.

Many people experience a range of emotions when finding out they have diabetes, including fear, sadness, guilt, and resentment. To deal with these feelings, they may deny the existence of the problem, trying not to think about it and hoping it will somehow just go away. They often continue to eat and behave just as they did before they received the diagnosis. They may forbid friends and family from commenting or admonishing them on their behavior. Not surprisingly, this behavior often leads to out-of-control blood sugars, and, depending on the length of the denial, damage to blood vessels or organs. When this damage comes to light, it is often accompanied by more fear, sadness, guilt, and resentment, which then makes the situation feel even more intolerable. This pattern is not uncommon in diabetes, and it is a cycle that keeps the person with diabetes stuck and unable to really manage their disease.

This book is about a way out of that struggle. It has been written to help you identify when this cycle is occurring and to help you find a working solution. Many self-help books on a variety of topics, including diabetes, will seek to help you find ways to reduce or eliminate the fear, sadness, guilt, and resentment you experience, operating from the belief that if we can take these feelings out of the cycle, there will be nothing to deny, and the problem will be solved. In essence, most approaches attempt to use fear as a motivator and then coach you to get rid of the fear so that it doesn't get in the way of managing your diabetes.

What such an approach forgets, though, is that diabetes *is* something to feel fear, sadness, guilt, and resentment about. We wouldn't dream of telling you that you should not feel these feelings about your diabetes, because diabetes is scary—it often represents a loss that any normal person would feel sad about. It involves making choices that you feel guilty about, and it's completely natural to feel resentful from time to time about being on a strict diet that others around you don't have to follow. So, instead of talking you out of your natural feelings or telling you to try to correct them the way you would correct high or low blood sugar, the purpose of this book is to help you find a way to *have your feelings and still take care of your diabetes.*

"But wait," you may say, "if I feel all these feelings, I will surely be swallowed up by them, and be rendered useless in the management of my diabetes!" This belief implies that your feelings are the only cause of your behavior. It also implies that if the feelings are overwhelmingly bad enough, you will have no choice but to do everything in your power to avoid them, even if it means avoiding your diabetes altogether. Throughout this book we will focus on the task of having these feelings as they occur and not allowing them to have power over your ability to take care of your diabetes.

The Acceptance and Commitment Therapy Approach

This book is based on acceptance and commitment therapy (ACT), an innovative approach to the struggles that human beings face. This approach, created by Dr. Steve Hayes and his colleagues (Hayes, Strosahl, and Wilson 1999), attempts to help people accept the difficult thoughts and feelings they have been attempting to avoid. The therapy targets this avoidance of thoughts and feelings, rather than the feelings or thoughts themselves, in order to help people make valued life choices.

"What does that mean?" you may ask. Well, in essence, an ACT approach to diabetes focuses on a diabetes-related version of the Serenity Prayer used in a variety of self-help and support groups around the globe: "Grant me the serenity to accept the things I cannot change, the courage to change the things I can, and the wisdom to know the difference." We will walk you through the complex task of learning how to accept difficult thoughts and emotions when they are there, while changing the things you *do* have control over—your behavior, and specifically such behaviors as exercising, eating a diabetes diet, taking medications or insulin if required, and monitoring your blood glucose—so that you can live a long and vital life with diabetes.

How This Book Came About and How to Use It

The kernels of this book were formed a number of years ago when we began using this approach with an amazing group of people with type 2 diabetes receiving care for their diabetes at a low-income health care clinic in the San Francisco Bay Area. These men and women were all in difficult situations, with unemployment, child care and family difficulties, transportation problems, and poverty all complicating the already complex task of managing their diabetes. They came from incredibly diverse cultural backgrounds and had a wide range of beliefs about both their diabetes and how they should handle their feelings about their diabetes. We began our work examining the usefulness of ACT with these individuals because we believed that if we could help them accept and manage their diabetes with all of the other forces at work in their lives, then we really had something.

And had something we did. Although the study we conducted was modest, and more research needs to be done, we found that many of our patients improved their blood sugar dramatically within three months and reported higher levels of exercise, diet, and blood-testing behavior than people given standard education about their diabetes (Gregg et al., forthcoming). They reported having many feelings and thoughts about their diabetes but still had better rates of self-management than they did before they encountered our training. This felt particularly important when we considered that in the time it had taken us to conduct the study, diabetes had gone from being the seventh leading cause of death in the United States to the sixth.

The urgency to share this approach with as many people with diabetes as possible felt even stronger.

In reading this book, we hope that you will have an experience similar to that of the patients in our studies, as well as the countless other people with diabetes we have treated over the years. We have learned immensely from their wisdom and have structured this book as a road map for you to use in order for you to benefit as well.

In order to get the most out of it, we recommend that you try a couple of things as you read this book. For starters, it's a good idea to have a diabetes journal or a notebook to help you keep track of things and write them down in one place as you read. This is not only so that you can jot down things that feel especially important that you want to remember, but also because there are many exercises and individualized planning tools available in this book and it's helpful to have all of your answers and objectives listed in one place. Remember, this is an approach to diabetes care that is based on a specific way of relating to your thoughts and feelings, so in order to best take advantage of this introspective approach, you will need to do a fair amount of writing about those thoughts and feelings.

In addition, we recommend that you talk about the ideas in this book and your plans for your diabetes care with people in your life. This sharing can help clarify some of the concepts, as well as give you as much support as possible for living an amazing life with diabetes.

Part I

Where We Start

CHAPTER 1

What Is It About Diabetes?

Henry is a fifty-nine-year-old married man who just found out that he has developed type 2 diabetes. Until recently, he worked for a computer company, but he had been feeling so low and tired lately that he decided to take early retirement and enjoy his golden years with his wife. Upon finding out about his diabetes diagnosis, Henry immediately thought of his father, who had died many years before. His father had spent the last of his years with terrible foot and leg pain and poor eyesight as a result of diabetes and had never managed to control his blood sugar. He had eventually died from a stroke that resulted from his diabetes. The thought of having the same fate was nearly too much for Henry to bear, and he sank into a serious depression. He would not leave the house, he stopped doing things he used to enjoy, and he would say things like, "What does it matter? This diabetes will kill me the same way it killed my father."

Henry's wife finally got him to go to the doctor, to talk about what he needed to do to treat his diabetes and to see what he could do to cope with it. His doctor gave him medication, advised him that he should exercise regularly, test his blood sugar often, and eat a diet low in sweets, salt, and fats. She also told him that he should try to not experience high levels of stress or depression—that these had been shown to have a relationship to high blood sugar and should be avoided. Upon hearing this, Henry tried hard not to think about his diabetes, given that it was stressful to him, and promised his doctor that he would try not to get too upset, sad, or angry.

Diabetes Is Hard

Henry's situation is not unique. Due to the causes of diabetes (which we discuss in chapter 2), a diagnosis of diabetes is often met with memories of loved ones who have suffered at the hands of the disease, shame and guilt at having gained too much weight, or fear about what the diagnosis may mean to the quality and length of one's life.

In addition, after the initial diagnosis, people with diabetes are instructed to become instant "health nuts"—eating a diet that is difficult for anybody to follow, exercising regularly, and keeping a constant eye on blood glucose to prevent it from getting too high or too low. Behaving in this way can be difficult enough, but for many people with type 2 diabetes, the diagnosis is given after years of not engaging in these behaviors. Only a small percentage of individuals diagnosed with type 2 diabetes report engaging in regular exercise or diet management before developing diabetes (Tuomilehto et al. 2001). Thus, not only do you have to adopt a complex and difficult new routine, but many of you will have to adopt it after a long period of not having had a regular fitness routine in place.

Diabetes Comes with a Range of Emotions

Like Henry, many people feel overwhelmed by their initial diagnosis, and this feeling may last for months or years. And why shouldn't it? Being told that you have a lifelong condition that can contribute to many different types of health problems *is* overwhelming. Even more overwhelming, for most people, is the enormous responsibility put on a person with diabetes by the rest of the story: that you alone can prevent this disorder from disabling or killing you, but in order to do so you have to radically change your relationship with food, exercise, stress, and your body, taking on a self-care regimen that is incredibly difficult, if not impossible, to carry out. Being told that you have a possibly life-threatening disease is overwhelming; having all the responsibility for preventing that with nearly impossible lifestyle changes is often crushing.

While everybody's experience is a little different, our patients have reported a number of feelings over the years. Below is a discussion of common reactions.

Fear

Whether it is a fear of needles, fear of fingersticks, fear about complications such as blindness or strokes, or fear of this disease taking your life, many people experience fear upon finding out about their diabetes. The symptoms that first appear when you have diabetes, such as feeling shaky or light-headed, or feeling as though something is wrong with your body, can be scary. In addition, the fear of hypoglycemic events (problems related to low blood sugar) is a common occurrence for people with diabetes. While this fear feels overwhelming, being afraid is a normal part of having this disease and does not indicate that something is wrong with you for feeling it.

Anger and Resentment

Like fear, anger and resentment are common elements for many people adjusting to life with diabetes. In fact, there may be some relationship between experiences of anger and the development of diabetes in some people. This may be because stress and anger can prevent you from taking proper care of yourself, which can lead to diabetes, or because the effects on the body of getting angry and upset produce a chemical chain of events that results in diabetes in some people (Vitaliano et al. 2002).

In finding out that one has diabetes, resentment is a feeling many people experience and few wish to admit. The experience of watching the world eat fast food and baked goods all around you, both in advertisements and real life, while being told that you—seemingly only you—cannot have these foods, is difficult for many people to bear without some resentment.

Guilt

One important aspect of diabetes, particularly type 2 diabetes, is the responsibility people feel for developing it. Diabetes, more than many other diseases and ailments, seems to be regarded as the fault of the sufferer, or as a disease caused only by one's behavior. This is often not the case, as we'll discuss in chapter 2, but the guilt and shame caused by the perception are very real emotions experienced by people with diabetes.

Sadness

Sadness is another common emotion experienced by people upon finding out they have developed diabetes. In our experience, sadness is many times what is left when all the other emotions are dealt with; diabetes and the threats it poses are often sad news to receive and a certain amount of grieving is a normal reaction to such sad news.

What Do *You* Feel?

Often it is difficult for us to take time to really think about how we feel about things that occur in our lives. It can be helpful to stop and think about what your experiences are, and particularly what feelings are there for us to work with.

One way to help understand your experiences is to put them down on paper. To do this, take a piece of paper or your diabetes notebook and a pen and write down what you felt when you found out you had diabetes (or were at risk for having it) and what other feelings have come along since that time. Have a hard time describing your feelings? Below are some common experiences. See if any of them fit and if so, add them to your list.

So How Do You Deal with These Emotions?

Most strategies for coping with difficult emotions attempt to help you deal with them so that they will go away. If you think about it, this is the way we all orient to things we don't want around—we try to eliminate, avoid, or at least control them. For example, if there is dirt on the floor that we don't want there, we vacuum it up. If we don't like the décor in a room, we change it. This is even true with people: we avoid people we don't like.

☐	Frustrated
☐	Sad
☐	Angry
☐	Guilty
☐	Relieved
☐	Ashamed
☐	Resentful
☐	Afraid
☐	Disappointed
☐	Stressed
☐	Regretful
☐	Anxious
☐	Peaceful
☐	Worried

Avoiding Thoughts

This strategy works incredibly well in most areas. One place it may not work as well, however, is with our thoughts. For example, try this exercise: For the next thirty seconds, do not think about a purple dragon (adapted from Hayes, Strosahl, and Wilson 1999). Don't think about its rough, scaly skin or the large toes on its curled feet. Don't think about its large nostrils, or its knotted spine, or its fiery breath. Don't think about its buggy eyes or its big heaving chest.

How did you do? Were you able to not think about a purple dragon for the whole thirty seconds? Chances are, the task was difficult, if not impossible. The reason for this is that the thought of a purple dragon, like many thoughts, cannot just be avoided, and even less so when the avoidance is purposeful. In fact, chances are, by trying *not* to think about one, you have now thought much more about purple dragons than you would have otherwise today. Trying not to think about a purple dragon automatically brings up thoughts about a purple dragon, if only just to remind you what you're not supposed to be thinking about.

Although it might seem obvious that you would have a difficult time forcing yourself to not think about something, this is exactly what many people do every day with foods forbidden from a diabetes diet. You may try not to think about chocolate cake so that you will be able to resist the temptation, but the act of trying to not think about it often makes thoughts of chocolate cake even more powerful than they would have been otherwise.

Avoiding Feelings

This is also the case with feelings like fear or anxiety. Suppose we told you that we had a very sensitive, state-of-the-art machine that we were going to hook you up to that would tell if you were at all anxious (Hayes, Strosahl, and Wilson 1999). And imagine we said your only task once you were hooked up to this machine would be to *not* be anxious. No matter what. You must remain relaxed, calm, and not worried. And we would know immediately if you were anxious, of course, because we would have you hooked up to this very sensitive machine. Do you think you could do it?

Many people would feel somewhat anxious simply at the thought that they are forbidden from feeling anxious. So what if we said that, in order to motivate you, we would put a gun to your head, and if you were anxious at all we would shoot you?

So how about this situation—do you think you would be anxious? Again, most people would not be able to help becoming anxious if they had to try hard not to be anxious, and certainly if somebody was "motivating" them with a firearm. This is because *not* being anxious is something to be anxious about. Said another way, if it is important that you don't feel stress, fear, or anxiety, you are more likely to feel just those emotions. Essentially, you experience stress about it being important that you not be stressed. Or shame about not being able to control your stress, sadness, anger, or guilt. Trying to avoid emotions often leads to more of that emotion, or whole new emotions.

And there is more to base this on than just your experience; a lot of research has been done that shows the same thing you just discovered—that trying to avoid thoughts and feelings tends to bring them even more powerfully than if you had not tried to avoid them. Studies have shown that not only are you *more likely* to have thoughts and feelings you try to avoid or suppress, but also that they will be of higher intensity than if they were not suppressed (Clark, Ball, and Pape 1991).

Is There Another Way?

Yes. Thankfully, there is another way. Although we typically try to protect ourselves from our emotions and thoughts, as discussed above, this often only serves to strengthen them, to make them more "sticky" and have a bigger role in our lives (Hayes, Strosahl, and Wilson 1999). With emotions, the alternative is to move *into* our feelings, rather than away from them. For many people, this is a rather unsettling idea that is accompanied by the belief that the feelings will become overwhelming if not managed appropriately. While we all have this belief from time to time and it is very convincing, it is generally not the case, and it often prevents us from really living our lives.

With thoughts the alternative is to step back and learn just to notice them mindfully, taking whatever might be valuable in them, and leaving the rest to play on as one might a loud radio in the next apartment (Hayes, Strosahl, and Wilson 1999). Learning to just notice thoughts is difficult to do, particularly when they are the really scary thoughts that sometimes come with diabetes. The solution is to develop these "just noticing" skills so well that you can use them even with things that are really frightening. The rest of this book will help you lay out a plan to help you take care of your diabetes, and live a vital life, while having your feelings and thoughts.

Summing It Up

Diabetes is a hard disease to have and to deal with, and many difficult emotions and thoughts come along with it.

Trying to avoid these thoughts and emotions often makes dealing with both them and your diabetes more difficult.

CHAPTER 2

The Basics:
Introducing Diabetes

Coping with diabetes is different than coping with other, less chronic illnesses. Diabetes requires that the majority of the day-to-day management be carried out by the patient him- or herself. From radical diet changes to blood testing or injections, the traditional medical role is performed not by the physician or nurse, but by the patient in their home, every day.

So why is that so difficult? Millions of people around the world with diabetes are taught the basics about diabetes and carry out these skills every day. The skills are not actually terribly difficult to learn and do. Rather, the difficulty with diabetes and maintaining good health lies not in the skills themselves, but that each of the skills requires a degree of motivation, coping, and consistency that is hard to muster, let alone maintain on a daily basis.

That's right—daily. One of the important things to remember with diabetes is that to prevent complications, you need to stay on track consistently. This requires a focus on living every day to its fullest, one day at a time. Helping you do that is our goal.

Goals of This Chapter

This chapter is really our way of saying "Let's introduce you to diabetes." If you already feel you have some good knowledge here, we invite you to keep reading, just for a refresher. If you aren't really sure if what you know is accurate, then we strongly encourage you to keep on reading. There are a lot of misconceptions about diabetes, and our goal is to try to present this information to you as clearly as we can. We want you to have some basic understandings here that will be important for the rest of our discussion in the book.

Warning: Potentially Overwhelming Information Ahead

Now, we do offer one word of caution. This information can get pretty overwhelming—and it's completely normal to feel that way. Not only is there a lot of information here, and for some of you, lots of new vocabulary terms, but some of the material may seem kind of scary. As we discussed in chapter 1, it's perfectly natural for you to have those feelings. Who wouldn't? The trick is to go ahead and have those feelings of worry, of frustration, of whatever you have—and keep on reading.

We invite you to go through the chapter at your pace. If you need to read ahead a little, and it still makes sense, come back to this material as soon as you can. If you want to read just a little at a time so that you understand the material here, do that. Remember, too, that there are many, many books available to you on diabetes and particularly on diabetes complications, which for many people are the overwhelming part of what we discuss in this chapter. The focus of this book is on helping you cope with and accept your diabetes and your thoughts and feelings about it. Books that have their primary focus on educating you about diabetes will be much more detailed and may be very helpful. The information here is meant to help you be able to understand the basics so that you can create your own individual plan for successful living with diabetes. We encourage you to seek more information and read other books that will help you understand the disease as much as you feel is helpful to you.

What Is Diabetes?

Still reading? Great!

The term *diabetes* actually refers to a group of diseases characterized by the body's difficulty generating or responding appropriately to *insulin*. Insulin is a hormone generated in an organ called the *pancreas*. The pancreas allows the sugar, called *glucose*, extracted from the foods we eat to be used by the cells and muscles. Our cells and muscles really need insulin. Essentially, insulin is like a key that unlocks the door to the cells and muscles so they can get the energy, the glucose, they need to function.

When the body does not produce or respond effectively to insulin, the cells and muscles do not get the energy they need, and the blood becomes full of this extra glucose. When the blood becomes full of glucose, the extra blood sugar coats all of the organs, tissues, and nerve fibers that come in contact with the blood. Over time, this causes damage to those blood vessels, organs, and tissues.

To picture how this damage occurs, let's imagine something. Imagine dipping a piece of thin cheesecloth first into a bowl of pure water. Let the cloth dry, and it is just the same as it was before. Now imagine taking that thin piece of cheesecloth and dipping it into a mixture of sugar and water and letting the cheesecloth dry. You probably know what would happen. You would soon have a stiff cloth board. If you bend it or twist it, it would quickly break.

Now imagine instead of cheesecloth, we did the same thing with the very delicate blood vessels and nerves (tiny fibers, really) that make up parts of your body. When the extra glucose is not allowed to enter the cells and muscles because there isn't enough insulin or the body is not effective at using it, that sugar hangs around in these blood vessels and nerve fibers over time. You can probably guess what happens, then, to the tiny fibers and blood vessels. Much like the thin cheesecloth, they become less flexible and get damaged. What happens when this damage occurs, specifically, is talked about later in this chapter.

Which Type of Diabetes Do You Have?

Whether a body does not produce insulin or simply does not respond effectively to the insulin it has is what determines which type of diabetes is diagnosed. A type 1 diabetes diagnosis typically means that the pancreas does not produce insulin or does not produce enough of it to do the job. Type 2 diabetes, on the other hand, normally means that there is plenty of insulin, but the body resists it for some reason. Type 1 diabetes used to be called "juvenile onset" or "insulin-dependent" diabetes, and type 2 used to be called "adult onset" or "non-insulin-dependent" diabetes, but there have been many cases of adults acquiring type 1 or children acquiring type 2. Not only that, but many individuals with type 2 diabetes inject insulin to control their blood sugar, so the old labels were scrapped and now we talk about them in terms of types.

How Did You Get Diabetes?

Often when people find out they have diabetes, the first thing they wonder is how they got it, quickly followed by how they can un-get it! How diabetes develops depends largely on what type of diabetes a person has.

Type 1 Diabetes

Type 1 diabetes is typically an *autoimmune disorder*, meaning that for some reason, your body thinks that there is a foreign invader in the pancreas and destroys the cells that produce insulin. Whether or not your body develops this autoimmune disorder is largely thought to be genetic (Jahromi and Eisenbarth 2006). This means that with type 1 diabetes, there's typically not a lot that can be done to cause or to prevent the onset of diabetes. Although a way to prevent it has not yet been found, all is not lost. There are many treatment options for individuals with type 1 diabetes, and with good management, more and more people with this diagnosis are living long, healthy lives.

Type 2 Diabetes

Type 2 diabetes, as we mentioned above, typically involves plenty of insulin, but there is a reduction in the body's ability to use it effectively. This state, called *insulin resistance*, may be caused by genetics, obesity, or a pancreas worn out from trying to work with an ineffective insulin system. The good news, if we can use that term, is that type 2 diabetes is dramatically affected by changing what you do—what you eat, how you exercise, and even how you think and feel. This type of diabetes is far more common around the world: type 2 diabetes is about ten times more common than type 1 (Centers for Disease Control and Prevention 2005). Because of this, most of the examples in this book are from individuals with type 2 diabetes, although the principles of self-management and coping we talk about generally apply to both type 1 and type 2.

Glucose and Hemoglobin A1c: The Numbers Game

There are two numbers that are important for you to know in managing your diabetes. The first is your glucose value. Earlier, we described glucose in the context of insulin and the importance glucose has in providing energy to your body. Glucose values are taken with a fingerstick and use a small drop of blood. These tests are typically done by you at home, and they provide information about the effects of different elements on your blood glucose levels. The second number is your hemoglobin A1c (HbA_{1C}) value. This is also determined by examining your blood, but this value is generally calculated from a blood draw by your doctor or diabetes clinic.

Glucose

Glucose values are measured in milligrams per deciliter, abbreviated "mg/dL." The range of these numbers is typically between 90 and 220. The numbers can go above and below this range, but that will indicate problems. Keeping your glucose values between 90 and 150 is generally the goal for diabetes management. "How do you do this?" Don't worry—we'll get to that.

Testing Glucose

Testing blood glucose levels is primarily done by you, the patient, at home with a glucose meter, and is typically done either daily or on a regular basis ranging from every other day to up to five or more times a day, depending on where you are in your diabetes management and the type of medication or insulin you take.

Although most people with diabetes are familiar with the use of their glucose meter and how to use it, there are a few things worth mentioning here with respect to testing glucose at home. First, it's important to use your glucose meter as a tool to study your body's individual response to different things you can do to impact your diabetes. This means that testing should not only be consistent from day to day, but also should be used before and after eating certain types of foods or engaging in certain activities so that you can better understand how *your* body is impacted by these things.

Another consideration when talking about blood glucose testing is the fact that many people don't want to use their glucose meter because fingersticks can be painful or uncomfortable. While strategies such as performing the fingerstick on the side of the finger, rather than on the pad, can sometimes minimize some of the pain, it is still not a painless procedure. It is perfectly normal to dislike this part of diabetes management and very understandable to avoid doing glucose testing in order to avoid this pain. Like many aspects of diabetes management, these uncomfortable feelings and resistance (and how you deal with them) are crucial to your overall diabetes management. Thus, the strategies described in the rest of this book will help you deal with these reactions and still monitor your blood glucose in order to take care of your diabetes.

Blood Glucose Values and What They Mean

The important thing to know about glucose numbers is that they will fluctuate quite a bit. We are really aiming for an average of 90 to 150. That is, if you have one reading at 90, one at 120, and another at 150, then your average is 120. One test and one result for blood glucose will not tell you enough about how well you are managing your diabetes. We'll say this another way: one fingerstick will not give you all of the information you need. The good thing about that is, if you are way out of the target range for one reading, it doesn't mean that your diabetes is out of control overall. The bad news, though, is that if you're in the right blood glucose range one day or at one reading, it also doesn't mean that you are always there.

One way to think about this is to use a camera as an example. A camera takes one picture of what has just occurred, a snapshot of those events. If you think about pictures of yourself that you have seen, some of them really capture you. But some of the photos might have not been what you think is a good picture of you—even though it *is* you in the picture. A blood glucose test is like this, too. It is a snapshot (so to speak) of your blood glucose at that moment in time. Just like with a photo, sometimes this value will be reflective of what is typically going on with your blood, and sometimes it will be higher or lower than is typical for you.

Now let's change the example to a movie camera. A movie camera can reflect more than what just occurred in that one moment in time. It gives us a view of what has occurred over a range of time, say an hour or even more. Blood glucose testing cannot really tell us this type of information. These values can change even in an hour! With diabetes, we want to know how you are doing over time, not just moment to moment. We can average blood glucose values, but another way to tell how you are doing over time is to measure something called hemoglobin A1c.

Hemoglobin A1c and Diabetic Control

Hemoglobin A1c (or HbA_{1C}) gives us a view of how your blood sugar has been over the past several months. This shows what we call *diabetic control* or, sometimes, a lack of control. As mentioned above, this test is typically conducted by a doctor or a lab, and results are given to you later. The values you see with hemoglobin A1c are in percentages. Although everybody is different, and you should talk with your doctor about the best range for you, the range of percentages we typically aim for with diabetes are between 4 percent and 6 percent, since these are typically the values found in people without diabetes and thus represent the least amount of risk for developing complications. Values higher than 8 percent are associated with more complications and disability. According to the American Diabetes Association, a value of 7 to 8 percent suggests something should be done to help.

Generally, getting a result for HbA_{1C} less than about 6.5 percent tells us that you have been doing a very good job managing your diabetes and that you are much less likely to develop the complications we discuss below. This percentage is roughly the same as an average blood glucose of 150, as can be seen in the figure on the next page.

Another way to think about glucose and hemoglobin A1c values is to use an analogy to baseball. Picture in your mind a baseball player hitting a home run. The crowd cheers, and that player just had a good day. Is he or she a good batter? Right then we can say he or she was for sure. Is he or she typically able to hit the ball this well? That's another question, and one we would need to know the batting average to answer.

What are glucose and hemoglobin A1c values in this example? The single time the ballplayer hit the ball at that time at bat is his or her glucose value in our example. This is a measure of how much glucose is in the blood at that moment. A home run for us with glucose values might be less than 120. Does it mean that the person with diabetes is always hitting "home runs"? Of course not. Just as with the baseball player, we don't need to always hit it out of the park to be doing well generally. Sometimes we swing and miss the ball, and sometimes we hit it. With diabetes that means sometimes you are

HbA1c and Blood Glucose Values

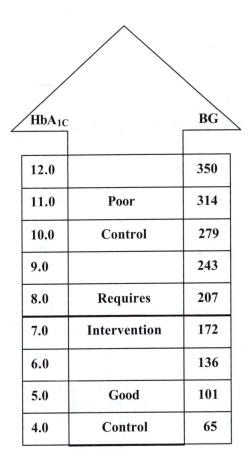

HbA$_{1C}$		BG
12.0		350
11.0	Poor	314
10.0	Control	279
9.0		243
8.0	Requires	207
7.0	Intervention	172
6.0		136
5.0	Good	101
4.0	Control	65

in your target range and doing very well, and sometimes you do not do as well. Still, if you are a baseball player, to have a good batting average, you need to hit the ball more often than not. To be in good diabetic control, you need to be in our appropriate glucose range more often than not. The HbA$_{1C}$ value tells us our "batting average" for glucose. It gives us a running average of sorts for how often you are in control of your diabetes, which really means preventing problems from developing.

As you can guess, we are aiming for more home runs, but no one expects a Babe Ruth or Barry Bonds here. There will be people you meet who are exceptional at keeping in good diabetic control. We are aiming for good values for glucose and hemoglobin A1c as often as we can. Our fans that help us celebrate are our friends and family. The great reward for having good diabetic control is our health and happiness. The result of having a poor batting average—poor diabetic control—is diabetes complications.

Complicated Complications

Whether your diabetes resulted from a lack of insulin or an ineffective batch of it, it is important to remember that there is nothing necessarily dangerous or fatal about diabetes itself. Having prolonged or significantly high or low blood sugar is the culprit in many of the problems we associate with diabetes: vision loss, amputations, kidney problems, nerve damage, heart disease, or even death. The goal of prevention is pretty straightforward: Keep blood sugar in the range of people without diabetes, and you lower your risk to about the same as theirs.

Here's the problem, and we bet you can say it to yourself before we tell you. These complications, well, they are really complicated sounding. Words like retinopathy, nephropathy, neuropathy—they all run together in a jumble of syllables all ending in something that sounds terrible. They are complicated-sounding words, and they are bad for you. That's the other problem. When most people hear words like these, as much as you want to keep listening (or reading), and as much as you know you need to keep listening (and keep reading), you just tune out.

This stuff is overwhelming.

Well, take a deep breath, because we are going to get through this together. We are going to try to make this information as simple as we can; and remember, the whole rest of this book focuses on using tools to deal with feelings and thoughts about what we discuss here. The reason you are being introduced to these health topics now is that you will develop the coping skills as you go through the book to deal with these very problems.

You Are In Charge!

Remember that you are in charge of this disease. The occurrence of these problems is not a foregone conclusion for your diabetes. Managing your blood sugar and moving in the direction of taking care of yourself and your diabetes will often allow you to keep these complications out of your experience.

Okay, so you're still reading and even rereading this material—good for you! Let's tackle the bodily complications first. The main parts of the body that can be affected by diabetes are your eyes, your nerves, your heart, and finally your kidneys. Each of these parts of your body has fancy medical names that go with them. The names are worth knowing even though they can seem sort of scary. The names are simply relating to the technical terms for the organs and parts of the organs that have problems. Using these names with your health care provider and doctor can really help them know that you understand what you're talking about. And when you don't really understand certain things, the terms can be a way to invite your care provider into a discussion with you.

A real trick to understanding these names is to know a piece of each word that several share in common, "pathy." The suffix or added part of the word, *pathy*, simply means that something is sick or has a problem. For example, if we take a word for a bodily organ and add "pathy" to the end, it will indicate that the organ has a problem. The challenge here is that few of the organ words are the ones that we typically use. Eye problems are not called "eyepathy." As you will see, we need to be more specific about the part of the eye that has a problem.

Retinopathy: The "Eyes" Have It

For your eyes, we will talk about the important part of the eye that allows you to not only see but to understand what you are seeing. This is the *retina*. The retina is a huge collection of tiny nerves that allow you to sense color and light in the world around you. These cells are supplied by a lot of blood in equally tiny vessels to help your eye continue to do what it's supposed to do. When the retina has problems we call it "retinopathy" (pronounced ret-in-op-athy).

Retinopathy, or *diabetic retinopathy*, happens when some of the blood vessels in your eyes are not getting the blood (and the oxygen it carries) they need. When this happens, your eyes can't work as well and can be damaged, leading to vision loss. Your eyes will try to heal themselves sometimes, and normally this is a good thing. The problem is, when they try to heal themselves by growing more blood vessels, this increased number of vessels can get in the way of your vision and potentially lead to vision loss. What we really want here is to avoid this problem altogether.

As we will discuss in chapter 11, diabetic retinopathy is a complex issue and the most important thing you can do besides control your blood sugar is to get regular eye exams.

Nephropathy: You Gotta Be Kiddin' Me with These Kidneys

Your kidneys come in a matched set and sit behind your abdomen, one on each side of your spine. The kidneys' main task is to help your body maintain a balance of important minerals like sodium and potassium. They help clear your body of harmful by-products from things you have digested, too. Another important job for the kidneys is to make the hormones that ultimately get red blood cells to the rest of your body. As you can see, the kidneys are very, very important.

Maybe it's because they are so important that they have so many complicated names. You will hear about the kidneys in relation to what is called "renal function," and importantly for us, *nephropathy* (pronounced nef-rah-pathy) or *diabetic nephropathy*. Diabetic nephropathy is a technically accurate way of saying kidney disease related to diabetes. Other things can cause kidney disease, too, but we will focus on how it relates to diabetes.

Part of what can happen with diabetes is frequent urinary tract infections. A lot of infections can cause the kidneys to become diseased. Another thing that can happen with kidney problems and diabetes is nerve damage. When there is nerve damage to the kidneys, it can ultimately lead to problems with emptying the bladder. This, too, can lead to infections.

When there is damage to the kidneys, ultimately it can be permanent and even fatal. While this is scary to think about, remember that these complications are often treatable in early phases and can often be prevented altogether. As with all of the complications discussed here, the key is to keep your body healthy and blood glucose in control.

Neuropathy: This Is All Getting on My Nerves

Running throughout your body is a complex system of nerves. These nerves send signals to your brain and receive signals to tell you what to do. They are absolutely essential to survival. Your nervous system can help you relax, and it can get you ready to run as fast as you can in times of danger. Your nerves help you feel the difference between rough sandpaper and the finest silk. They can tell you when you feel a soft breeze on your face, and they can tell you when you have a rock in your shoe.

As much as we need nerves, it may surprise you to find that this is one of the hardest-hit parts of our body with diabetes. We don't know exactly how nerves are damaged with diabetes, but they are. It could be related to blood supply to the nerves (like with the eyes in retinopathy), or it could be related to blood sugars damaging these very, very small cells. The bottom line is that damage to the nervous system can have extreme effects on your survival. The area of medicine studying nerves is called *neurology*. The key to this word is the root "neuro," meaning nerves. Damage to the nervous system is called *neuropathy* (pronounced ner-op-athy).

When nerve damage occurs in your body, you may feel tingling sometimes, pain at other times, and sometimes you don't feel anything at all. This can lead to huge problems. For instance, imagine that you step on a tack. This really hurts! Your body is telling you, "Hey! Get this out of my foot!" When you feel the pain, you look at your foot, remove the tack, and treat the wound. If it keeps hurting after a few days and looks red, you make sure you don't have an infection. The nerves in your foot are constantly giving you feedback about what is going on down there.

Now imagine you step on a tack, but the nerves at the bottom of your foot aren't working properly. They don't send a signal of pain to your brain to tell you something is wrong. This means (you guessed it) the tack stays in. Even if it falls out, or if you felt enough to take the tack out, you may not feel what is happening down there with the development of an infection. If an infection continues on the foot, it can spread. This can ultimately lead to massive infection and even amputation.

If you take the time to look at the bottoms of your feet, you could see this process happening. Most of us aren't accustomed to looking at the soles of our feet very often, but this is a very important task for people with diabetes!

Even though we have been focusing on nerves for the feet, remember what we just said about your nervous system running through your whole body. These nerves go to your hands, your fingers, your toes, your eyes, and important systems that control blood pressure, digestion, heart rate, and even sexual functioning. The consequences of nerve damage can affect all of these areas, as we discuss in more detail in chapter 11.

Cardiovascular Disease: Taking It All to Heart

We probably don't need to tell you how important your heart is. Doctors refer to it with the term "cardio." You know it is responsible for pumping all the blood you need throughout your body, taking oxygen to all of the cells that need it to survive. You probably know that your larger blood vessels, called your *vascular system*, need to be in good working order to get that blood from the heart to where it needs to go. This larger set of blood vessels is referred to as *macrovascular* (*macro* meaning bigger) as opposed to the smaller blood vessels like those in the eye that we discussed briefly above called *microvascular*.

The problems that can develop with diabetes that involve the heart and vascular system are called *cardiovascular disease* and *macrovascular* or *microvascular complications*. These complications are some of the most common problems people with diabetes eventually develop. Of course, lots of people without diabetes develop cardiovascular disease, too. In fact, this is the number one killer of all Americans each year (Rosamond et al. 2007).

That said, the risk of heart problems is one of the biggest threats people with diabetes face. Cardiovascular problems are related to heart attacks, stroke, and other health problems. It is essential that you stay on top of your health, as these complications can largely be prevented with an improved diet, lowered blood sugar, lowered cholesterol, and lowered blood pressure.

The other areas of the body we will talk about that can be affected by diabetes are much broader than those we just listed. They are complex behaviors and psychological events that require more discussion, but are equally important to the more physical complications discussed above.

Sexual Functioning: This Is Getting a Little Personal

Although we don't really like to talk about it publicly, sexual functioning is a very important part of being human. Whether it is for procreation and offspring, connecting to a loved one, or just having fun, when the sexual system no longer works as well, it means problems. Given the effects of diabetes on the circulatory system, many men and women with diabetes experience some form of *sexual dysfunction*. With males this typically means problems with sustaining an erection, and with females it's generally comprised of problems with lubrication for intercourse.

You may be saying to yourself, "That makes sense, given what I just read." The sex organs are filled with tiny blood vessels and nerve endings. If you develop problems with the nerves or blood vessels and they are damaged, this will affect the organs' ability to function. It can be just that simple.

There is nothing simple about sexual dysfunction though. Sexual intimacy in relationships is a complex social process. When there are physical problems in this area, it is not uncommon to find psychological and relationship problems. These problems can make this situation feel even worse. Feelings of anxiety and depression or sadness are common occurrences with problems of sexual functioning. With anxiety, many people are so worried that they may not be able to "perform" the way they want, sexual intimacy becomes a physical impossibility. It's not a mystery that some people with sexual dysfunction report feeling sad or depressed about their problems. With sadness and depression, it is fairly common to hear people report that their desire (or libido) has reduced a great deal, and they are just not interested in sex.

While there is a relationship between feeling depressed and reduced sexual functioning, it turns out that deep sadness is an issue for diabetes separate from sexual problems. Depression is a problem with diabetes all by itself.

Depression: When It All Gets You Down

All of the information in this chapter alone could get anyone feeling down. In fact, feeling sad and overwhelmed, feeling like you can't do anything about these issues, are all very normal reactions to being diagnosed with diabetes. There is an important distinction for us to make here about our feelings with respect to the word "depression." Feeling sad temporarily is often called "feeling depressed." That's a normal, everyday use of the term "depression." *Clinical depression* is a diagnostic term used by mental health and medical professionals to refer to a more long-standing problem than adjusting to very difficult news or feeling blue.

We are not trying to say that whatever sad feelings you are having aren't worthy of a label like depression. The key to understanding what professionals refer to as a diagnosis of clinical depression or *major depressive disorder* is that it is not just feeling down—it is feeling kept down. People diagnosed with clinical depression experience a variety of problems for two weeks or more, never feeling very normal or happy. These problems can include sadness, not getting pleasure from things, trouble sleeping, changes in appetite, lack of concentration, feelings of excessive guilt, feelings of fatigue, and even thoughts of suicide (American Psychiatric Association 2000). While most people feel sad, especially in response to dealing with diabetes, clinical depression does not happen to everyone.

Still, major depressive disorder is one of the most commonly diagnosed psychiatric conditions. Between 12 and 20 percent of the American population will be diagnosed with clinical depression during their lifetime (Hollon et al. 2005). Factors that impact depression include environmental challenges like coping with disease, disruptions in important relationships, and other life changes.

If you feel like you might be suffering from clinical depression (particularly if you are feeling suicidal), we encourage you to talk to your health care provider. He or she will discuss options with you that can help. If you believe that what you're struggling with is sadness in reaction to all of the life changes you are making or needing to make because of diabetes, well, you have come to the right place. This book is just for you. You will learn how to experience these natural feelings *and* take care of your diabetes *and* live a long and healthier life.

What Is the Effect of Good Diabetes Control?

Let's get back to the good news here. We discussed the importance of having good diabetic control in the section prior to the one on complications. Here we want to wow you a little with the research showing what we are talking about. This section is meant to help convince you that those problems we just talked about are actually often avoidable. In the last two decades a number of very big, very elaborate studies have been conducted with individuals with diabetes in order to better understand the relationship between diabetes, high glucose, and complications like vision loss, kidney problems, and heart disease.

The Diabetes Control and Complications Trial (DCCT)

The Diabetes Control and Complications Trial (1993) was a ten-year study conducted by the National Institute of Diabetes and Digestive and Kidney Diseases in the United States. In this study, 1,441 patients with type 1 diabetes were randomly assigned to either normal diabetes management or an "intensive" management condition. Intensive treatment involved testing glucose levels and administering insulin four or more times daily, strict diet and exercise regimens, and monthly visits to a physician, nurse educator, dietician, and behavior therapist.

The results of the study showed that patients in the intensive management condition had a 76 percent reduced risk for eye disease, a 50 percent reduced risk for kidney disease, and a 60 percent reduced risk for nerve disease. Intensive treatment also significantly lowered the risk of developing high cholesterol, which is a key factor in the development of heart disease.

Although our focus in this book is on type 2 diabetes, you can see that a focused management of glucose really changed people's lives in this study. The reduction in risk for eye, kidney, nerve, and heart disease is impressive!

UK Prospective Diabetes Study (UKPDS)

In a similar study examining individuals with type 2 diabetes, the UK Prospective Diabetes Study (1998) demonstrated similar results as the Diabetes Control and Complications Trial. The UKPDS was a twenty-year study examining the effects of intensive management on over 5,000 patients with type 2 diabetes in England, Northern Ireland, and Scotland. This study found that better glucose control reduces the risk of eye disease by 25 percent and early kidney damage by roughly 33 percent in individuals with type 2 diabetes.

The researchers also found that better blood pressure control in patients with high blood pressure reduces the risk of death from any of the long-term complications of diabetes, stroke, and vision problems all by about 30 percent. This study showed that the main medications used to treat diabetes (metformin, sulphonylureas, acarbose, and insulin) are all pretty equal in reducing high blood sugar, and that people who are overweight may benefit from some of these medications.

Knowledge Is Power, But We Need Something Else

Given all of the complicated and scary things we have discussed in this chapter, it is no wonder that many people with diabetes prefer not to think about their disease. Research consistently shows us that many people with type 2 diabetes are not successfully managing their disease with respect to blood sugar and hemoglobin A1c values. Researchers are just starting to realize what people with diabetes and diabetes doctors have known all along—that understanding how to take care of one's diabetes does not necessarily mean that a person will take care of their diabetes. This is not because the person with diabetes is weak or a failure. Taking care of one's diabetes requires lifestyle changes that are incredibly difficult to make and even more difficult to continue over time.

In the next chapter we will begin to explore why you want to take care of your body, your health, and manage your diabetes. With the understanding you have gained from this chapter, your doctor or health care provider, and other sources, we will teach you some skills to be able to do the things you need to do in order to live a healthier life.

Summing It Up

About 90 percent of people with diabetes have type 2 diabetes, which can often be managed with diet, exercise, medication or insulin, and careful monitoring of blood sugar.

There are many complications associated with poor control of your diabetes, but many of these are preventable.

Although education is important, it is important to tie the information to a focus on why you want to take care of your diabetes; that will be the focus of this book.

CHAPTER 3

Value Added

Now that we have discussed some of the basics of diabetes, it's time to take a closer look at what you want your life with diabetes to include. In some ways, this is the exact opposite of the hope that many people have that their diabetes will go away. This is about figuring out how to live an amazing life *with* diabetes.

Values as a Compass

Living an amazing life with diabetes starts with spending some time focusing on your values and goals. By *values*, we do not mean social or moral values that other people suggest you need to have, or values embraced because you would otherwise feel guilty. Instead, we're talking about what is most important to you because *you* assign them the most value or because they bring you joy. Your values are the elements of your life that give your life meaning, so when you are living in a way that is consistent with your values, you are living a full, meaningful life that is full of vitality.

One way to think about this is to think of your values as your own personal compass. When you pay attention to your compass, it helps guide you in the direction that you most want to go in your life and helps you live in a way that means the least amount of regret at the end of your life.

Values Compass

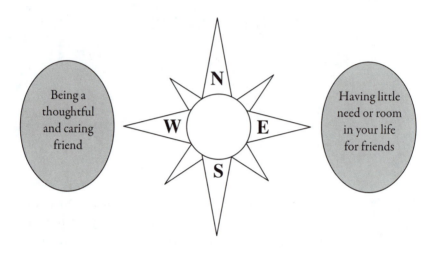

This values compass (Hayes, Strosahl, and Wilson 1999), like a real compass, only gives you a general direction such as north, south, east, or west. It doesn't tell you exactly which landmarks to pass on your way. In that way, paying attention to your values is sort of like looking at a compass to know that you are heading west: it is only a direction, not a destination, so you never are finished living your values and there is always more "west" to go. For example, if you have the value of wanting to be a thoughtful and considerate friend, you never actually complete that task—you can do many thoughtful and considerate things for your friends and still do more tomorrow to be a considerate friend, just like you could head west to California, and from there head west to Hawaii, and then from there west to Asia, and still have more "west" to go tomorrow.

Getting Started

To start this process, it is important that we first think about your life as a whole as it is right now. In fact, get your diabetes notebook or piece of paper and a pen, and let's take a second to write down some notes about your life.

Positively Fabulous

Let's start with the positives. What are you most proud of or pleased about? Write down the top two or three things that stand out. For some people it is the great kids they have raised or are raising, or the great job they do at work. For other people it's an amazing garden or a backhand tennis swing. Maybe this is a hard question for you to answer. If so, that's okay, and it gives us some really important information. It means we have an opportunity to create some areas in your life for you to feel proud of.

Challenge Time

So now that we have the list of positives, what stands out as a negative? When you think about your life, are there things that you wish were different? If so, jot down the one or two things that feel the biggest. For some people, the things that feel like negatives are things like a difficult relationship with a friend, family member, or coworker, or not being on track with their diabetes care. Try to think about each challenge as specifically as possible. For example, rather than writing down that your challenge is having diabetes, try to think about what exactly about having diabetes is most challenging for you. Is it the difficulties you have with taking care of yourself? Or is it the effects on your relationships? This will help us focus how we think about each challenge, rather than leaving us with something that is hard to do anything about. If no challenges come to mind, that's okay. The purpose of this is to acknowledge the biggest areas that we might work on, not to find problems.

Dream a Little Dream

Next we want to talk about your dreams and wishes related to your diabetes. Diabetes values are just like regular values, but for our purposes here we want to make sure that we spend some time focusing on your specific values in terms of your diabetes care. This is important because unlike some diseases, remember that diabetes involves a lot of active behavior on your part.

The question we want you to ask yourself at this point is: what would you want your life with diabetes to look like, if you could choose how you took care of your diabetes without any limitations? Here, don't list the realities of your diabetes management, but rather what you most wish your diabetes management would be described as. Although it is tempting to list as your dream that your diabetes would suddenly go away, we're more interested in how you would ideally describe *your care* of your diabetes, assuming it isn't going anywhere.

For example, if you dream of being the type of person who is very good at eating a diabetic diet and exercising while resisting the temptation to indulge in things that will send your blood sugar out of whack, go ahead and list that. Or, if you dream of being the type of person who is always on top of their medication and regularly tests and keeps track of their blood sugar ratings, write that.

Interestingly, we have found that the dreams people have about their relationships and activities are often directly related to their diabetes values. For example, when asked why it is important for them to take care of their diabetes, patients have told us time and again that it is important to them to have good health in order to be around for their family, or to attend a grandchild's graduation, or to remain an active person. These other values are directly related to what we would think of as "diabetes values" because there really is no distinction between the person with diabetes and their hopes and dreams for the future.

Down to the Nuts and Bolts: Defining Your Values

In order to use your values as a compass for the road ahead, we first need to spend some time defining what your individual values are. This is the hard part for some people.

Funeral Exercise

Knowing specifically how we'd like our life to look if we had a choice is a daunting task for even the most aware person. One exercise that is sometimes helpful is what we call the funeral exercise (Hayes, Strosahl, and Wilson 1999). In this exercise, we ask you to imagine that you are at your own funeral. Imagine that you can see all the people there and everything that is going on, but nobody can see you. Now, instead of imagining what everybody *would* say about you in this situation, we want you to imagine what you would most *want* everybody to be saying. We want you to dream really big here; try not to let the "realities" of the situation restrict you.

Husband/Wife/Partner

For example, first think about your husband, wife, or partner. If you don't have a partner but you want one, imagine the type of partner you would like to have. What would you want them, whether or not they currently exist, to say about you regarding what type of partner you were? Write down what you would wish for them to say (remember, this is what you would like them to say, not necessarily what they would say right now).

Family

Now think about your family. Among your family members (mom, dad, sisters, brothers, aunts, uncles, grandparents, cousins, nieces, nephews, sons, daughters), who would you like to speak at your funeral? What would you want each of them to say about what type of daughter/son/sister/brother/niece/nephew/grandchild/cousin/aunt/uncle/mom/dad you were? Write that down.

Note: Some of the people in these relationships may have passed away already, and thinking about what you wished you were in those relationships may feel uncomfortable or sad. While nothing can go back and change what characterized those relationships, noticing these feelings can be very helpful in determining what is most important to you in your existing relationships, which is why we're doing this exercise. We'll talk more in chapter 5 about dealing with feelings such as sadness and regret.

Friends

Next, think about your friendships. What type of friendships do you currently have? What kind of friendships do you wish you had? Do you like having many friends with whom you are social, or do you prefer to have a few close friends with whom you can share your inner experiences? Imagine who among your friends you would want to stand up and speak about what kind of friend you were. If you don't have a friend close enough that you can imagine them doing that, imagine what type of person you would like to stand up as your friend. What would you like them to say about what kind of friend you were? Write down what you would want them to say about you.

Work/Daily Activities/Education

Now imagine a representative from your work or where you spend your time during the day who would say something about what kind of an employee/boss/worker you were. Would you want them to say that you were conscientious, or relaxed and spontaneous, or driven and ambitious? Maybe you would want them to say all of these or none of these. How would you most want to be remembered for how you were as an employee/boss/worker? Write down what you would most want them to say.

And what would you want them to say about how you were with the people you worked with? Would you want them to say that you were always focused on the work at hand or that you were a fun coworker? Remember that this is not what they would necessarily say now, but what you would most wish for them to say about you if you could choose. Again, write their statements as you would want them to be.

Now imagine somebody standing up to talk about what kind of learner you were. What would you most like for them to say about how you learned and what you did regarding education and growth during your lifetime? Maybe you are currently a student. Would you want them to say that you were always learning, taking classes, and trying to expand your knowledge? Would you want them to say that your learning was more real-world, and that you found your experiences to be more valuable than what you could learn in a classroom? What adjectives would you want them to use, if you could choose them, about what type of learner you were?

Citizenship

Now imagine somebody from your community rising to say something about what kind of citizen you were. What would you want them to say? Would you want them to say that you were a respectful neighbor who minded their own business or that you were very involved in your community? Would you want them to say that you gave your time to causes that were important to you, and if so, which ones? Would you want them to say that you were involved in the political structure of your community, state, country, or world in order to bring about changes you believed in, or that you tried to make a difference in less political avenues? Write what you would want them to say about your citizenship.

Faith/Spirituality

If it applies, picture somebody who represents your faith or spiritual beliefs standing up to speak about your spirituality or religion. What would you want them to say? Maybe you would choose for them to say that you were a very religiously connected person who had a deep faith in God or their church structure. Maybe it would feel more consistent for them to say that you were connected to the earth or to your own spirituality in a way that was separate from organized religion. Check with your own spiritual values and write what you would choose for this type of representative to say about you, if anything.

Health

Finally, select a representative from your life to stand up and say what you would most want them to say about how you took care of your health. Would you wish for them to say that you were conscientious about your health and took good care of yourself always? Would you want them to say that you had a relaxed attitude about your health and that you always lived your life to the fullest, even if it was not always the healthiest? What would you want them to say about how you took care of your diabetes? Keep in mind, this is not necessarily what somebody would say about how you take care of yourself or your diabetes now, but what you would choose for them to say if everything in your life was going exactly how you wanted it to. Write down what they would say about your care of yourself and your diabetes.

Now that you have written down what you would want somebody to say about you in each of these domains, let's take some time to distill out a list of your values. Take a minute and look at what you would want people to say about you in each of the domains above. The information here is important, because your values for each of these domains are within what you have written. For instance, if you wrote that you wanted your closest friend to stand up and say that you were a thoughtful, caring, and loyal friend who was always fun to be around and who could be trusted with a secret, it means that you value being a thoughtful, caring, loyal, fun, and trustworthy friend. For each of the areas discussed above, look at what you wrote down, and generate one or two sentences describing your values for each area, just as we did with the friendship example. Don't forget that these statements should reflect your values, not what you think you should value or what other people think you should value.

Living Your Values: Real-Life Goals

As noted above, there are many reasons to spend some time thinking about where you would most want your life to be if you could control all of the variables. Perhaps most importantly for our purposes here, this assessment provides us with a clear direction in which to start to set some *goals*. Goals are similar to values in that they are direction points, but whereas we use values as a compass, goals are locations along the map that we are heading toward. Locations, unlike a direction like "west," can be reached and successfully checked off the list. Thus, goals are the points along the way to living a value-driven life (Hayes and Smith 2005).

In order to determine our concrete goals for this journey, we first need to look at what you've written down above concerning your values in all of the areas. What stands out as a theme? Do you notice that relationships play a central role in how you would choose to live your life? Do you notice that a particular style has emerged, like being laidback and relaxed or conscientious and ambitious? Write down the two or three patterns that you notice from the assessment above.

Romantic Relationship Goals

Now let's define the goals you have related to these values. First take a look at your relationships, if that was a pattern that stood out for you. Look first at your values about romantic relationships, if you listed any. If you currently have a partner and you listed things you would like to be more of in that relationship (thoughtful, loving, respectful, etc.), try to come up with one or two specific things you could do that would constitute living that value. For example, if you listed that you valued being a loving partner, what is one thing that you could do that would be loving toward your partner? Maybe you know that he or she would love to get a surprise "I was just thinking about you" note or phone call. Or maybe he or she would love a massage or an expression of your love and appreciation. The point here is not to come up with an idea that you think would be a loving gesture toward just anybody, but a loving gesture toward your partner in particular. In this vein, try to come up with two or three specific actions that you could do that would be in line with your values related to your romantic relationship. The actions can be big gestures, like taking your partner on a trip around the world, or small, like a phone call to let your spouse know you are thinking about them. Most people have a combination of small and large goals in all of the domains. The most important point is to make sure that the goals are achievable, whether short- or long-term, and are things that you can do or start doing today.

If you do not currently have a partner, it's still important to think about how you might go about living your values in this area. For example, if you listed that you value being a connected partner to somebody in the future and you are not currently in a committed relationship, it may make sense to evaluate any relationships you are in to see if you want to have committed romantic relationships with anybody currently in your life. If so, goals can be generated to move you in that direction. If there is nobody currently in your life with whom you wish to have a connected relationship but you value being in a committed romantic relationship, your goals might be related to things like joining interest or hobby groups, singles clubs, or an online dating service in order to find that special person. It should be noted that these types of steps sometimes cause an increase in discomfort or anxiety for some people, and that is perfectly okay. We'll talk about the things that get in the way of living these values below; for right now, our task is just to list what the goals would be.

Family Relationship Goals

Next, think about your values related to your family relationships. For many people, these relationships are the most difficult to navigate. If we stay focused on our values, however, it often becomes easier to see where to head with family relationships. For example, if you listed a value of being a caring son or daughter to a parent, what types of goals could we generate for that value? Maybe for your parent(s), one caring gesture would be a card or letter letting them know how much they mean to you. Or maybe, if they live near you, it would entail making a regular, monthly date for lunch or coffee. Again, these goals can be big or small, as long as they are actions you can take to live your values today.

If your parents are no longer living, or if you have more family, in-laws, or children, maybe your goals would be more focused on what type of sibling, cousin, in-law, or parent you can be. Again, the task is to look at what your values are and come up with specific goals related both to each value and to the specific person you are thinking of. If we pay attention, people in our lives will often tell us ways to be loving, respectful, caring, or patient with them.

Friendship Goals

Friendships are an important part of living a full life for many people. In examining your values related to friendships, what is most important to you? What might be some goals you could set in this area? If you value being a friend who is always there, maybe a goal would be to pick up the phone and see how your closest friends are doing, or to set up a time to get together. If you don't have as many friends as you'd like, maybe a goal would be to engage in activities, groups, or events that might bring you in contact with people with similar interests in order to increase your exposure to befriend-able people. Whatever your values for what type of friend you want to be, write down a few key things that would be in line with living them.

Employment and Daily Activities Goals

Now think about the values you listed related to being a worker/coworker. If you value being a conscientious worker, what are some particular things that you could do to be more conscientious than you are currently? Maybe you're already doing everything you can on this value, but if not, what are some steps that you could take? If you value being a loyal employee who helps your company or organization grow, spend a few minutes thinking about what specific goals you could have related to that value. For example, maybe a goal would be to attend meetings or trainings not typically required but that might help you gain a better sense of the organization and ways in which you might contribute. Or, if you value being a supportive, involved coworker, maybe a goal would be to organize an after-work get-together with your colleagues to broaden your understanding of them and their lives. If you work at home at a home business or as a full-time parent or homemaker, your work values and goals may be related to your family or parenting goals, or your values for what type of home environment you want to create.

If you do not currently have a job or are retired, it's important to still examine your values related to work, in that they may provide information about areas that are important to you that might not be as expressed now as they have been in the past. For instance, if you value contributing to the culture or helping people and you recently retired from a job in which that value was met, one goal might be to find a volunteer position that allows you to still contribute or help out. Or, if you value being a hard worker and you are currently unemployed, a goal may be to look for a temporary job while you are looking for a more permanent position in your field.

Education Goals

One value that is important to some people and not as important to others is in the area of education and learning. Take a look at the values you wrote down for learning, if any. What goals can be generated from those values? For example, if you value being a lifelong learner, what does that mean for you specifically? Maybe a goal would be to take a class at the local community center or community college in an area that you know nothing about but have always been interested in. Or maybe a goal would be to expand your own reading or learning through less formal means. If you value organized education, maybe a goal would be to go back to school for the degree or certificate you always wanted to obtain and never dedicated the time to. Your goals can be big, like obtaining a degree, or small, like checking a book out of the library on a subject you've always been interested in, as long as they are actions you can take each day to move in the direction of your values. Again, this value is not one that is important to everybody, but for some people it helps define how to incorporate their interests into their lives and futures.

Community Involvement Goals

Another value that is not important to everybody but is very important to some is the value of community involvement or citizenship. When you look at your values in this area, what do you see as possible goals? If you value being involved and volunteering your time but are not sure how to start, one goal might be to go to a volunteering website, such as www.volunteermatch.org, and find out what opportunities are available in your community. Or, if you value being part of the political arena and feel an affiliation with a political cause, party, or candidate, a goal might be to contact that organization and join a campaign.

Spiritual Goals

For some people, the most important of their values are their spiritual values. For others, these values either are lower down the list or do not apply at all. Whichever camp you fall into, look at the spiritual values for a minute. What goals can be generated to help bring this aspect of your life more into focus? If you value being connected to your spiritual source on a daily basis, one goal might be to set aside time every day for prayer, meditation, or reflection. If you value being a dedicated and loyal member of a religious community or congregation, a goal may be instead to dedicate a certain amount of time per week to attending services or volunteering for a congregational role. If this is not a value that holds a great deal of importance to you in your current life situation, is that something that you wish to be different? If so, a goal might be to spend time learning or exploring spiritual traditions or religions to determine what is the best fit for you.

Health Goals

Finally, we come to your health values. When you think about your values related to your health, what do you notice? Some people notice that thinking about setting goals for health-related values reminds them of times they have tried to set health goals and not been able to reach them. This can be very disappointing and may make it difficult to think about setting more. For our purposes here, let's start with just noticing what your values are. Do you value being a person who spends time on their health, or are other values more important for your time at this point? If you value spending time on your health, what types of goals rise to the top when you think about this value?

One example of what type of goal we are talking about might be to consistently eat two servings of vegetables per day, moving up from there. For some people, eating vegetables is not the difficult thing while getting daily exercise is more challenging. Other people find that regularly testing their blood sugar or taking medications is the difficult step. At this point, try to focus on what area of your health values needs the most help and set reasonable, obtainable goals in those areas without worrying too much about what has prevented you from making changes in these areas in the past. We'll talk about things that prevent us from living these values in a minute. But for now our task is to determine what "locations" you would stop at in your journey "west."

Barriers, Barriers, Barriers

Taking the time to sit down and think about what we value in a given area and what specific goals and actions might be called for in order to live those values are the important first steps in mapping out a direction for creating a meaningful life. However, these tasks purposefully leave out an important aspect of moving forward in that direction: the barriers to getting there. If there were no barriers to getting to these desired locations in our lives, you would already be there and probably would not have bothered to buy this book. In reality, there are barriers, and they often feel as real as a brick wall standing in your path. Let's take a few minutes and explore what types of barriers might be present in your life.

Time Barriers

A big obstacle for many people in attempting to move toward their values is time. There never seems to be enough time to get all of the things done that we'd like to, and many of the things that might enhance our lives end up feeling like extras that we just don't have time to even think about, let alone plan and execute. A patient once told us that taking the time to set goals and define values was like taking the time to teach a monkey how to rhyme; it was an extra that wouldn't matter because the monkey would never learn to talk. In the analogy, the patient was saying that it would never actually matter if he defined all of the things he wanted his life to include because a crucial element was missing: time to do them. He was too busy "putting out fires" and dealing with the negative consequences of what he hadn't yet finished or taken care of to make positive changes in his relationships and health behaviors.

This perspective is a common one and one that we all fall into. Unfortunately, this isn't how most of us would choose to live our lives. And yet, we are exactly the ones who end up taking on too much, or not setting limits, or not asking for what we need in order to have this life be important and meaningful. That is not to say that sometimes we don't all get behind; but if you only get to go through this life once, don't you want to balance those obligations with the things that really matter?

The process of finding time to live your values can be a difficult endeavor at first. It will require being choosy about which goals you focus on to begin with and learning to set limits on things that are not consistent with your values. This may take some time to balance, but once you get accustomed to thinking in terms of your values and goals, it will become easier to live your life in a way that creates time for things that really matter.

Energy Barriers

Another obstacle to living values that many people struggle with is finding the energy to engage in a whole new set of behaviors and activities. This may be particularly important for a person with diabetes, especially if their blood sugar is not in good control. If you find, as you set off to take steps toward living your values, that your energy is too low to follow through, it may be important to start with your health-related values first and make changes in your diet and exercise (see chapters 7 and 8 for detailed information on diabetes-related exercise and nutrition) to bring about a more energetic you.

Feeling Barriers and Thought Barriers

Finally, the last area of potential barriers to moving forward in the direction of your values may be your feelings and thoughts. Maybe thinking about a particular area of your life is overwhelming, and you can't stop thinking about it or you try to avoid thinking about it altogether. Maybe you feel sad, lonely, or anxious and try to push these feelings away. This is certainly one approach taken by many people, but as we discussed some in chapter 1, this tactic typically does not work long-term and may be what has prevented you from living your values to begin with.

Take the example of Ken, an overweight forty-five-year-old man with type 2 diabetes who was referred to our clinic by his doctor to get help finding the time and energy to manage his diabetes more effectively. It became clear pretty quickly that one major difficulty for Ken was that he was incredibly lonely and was preoccupied with worry that his diabetes would cause him to die without ever having had the opportunity to meet somebody, get married, and have a family. Because of this, and his feelings of shame about his body and his belief that nobody would want to be romantically involved with him because of his weight, he tried hard not to think about either his loneliness or his diabetes. Ken reported that he would go straight home from work and sit on the couch watching TV every evening to try to "numb out" these feelings. Not surprisingly, both his diabetes and his love life were not improving much from his couch.

In the next chapter we will spend some time talking about ways to cope with your feelings about your diabetes, as well as the other feelings that may be brought up by focusing on what's important in your life. It's important to remember, however, that while it may seem as though these feelings can stop you from heading in the direction of your values, at every point you are in the driver's seat and therefore you determine how far west you go.

For Your Fridge

Defining your own personal values is an important step in living a vital, meaningful life. This step, however, is not as useful when it serves as a one-time exercise as when it helps guide consistent, lifelong change. The way to ensure a more consistent change is to keep your values present with you on a day-to-day basis.

One easy way to bring this exercise into your life is to create a version of the lists you've made and ideas you formulated here to put in a central place in your home or living quarters. The best place for many people is on their refrigerator. We find that this works particularly well in the case of health-related values, but many people make a list of their values for all areas of their life, as well as the goals they are working toward, and post it on the refrigerator so that they are reminded of them every day. One patient of ours came up with this format for his list. It is adapted from a similar list in Hayes and Smith's *Get Out of Your Mind and Into Your Life* (2005, 186):

Value	Goals	Barriers	Solution
Being a loving, supportive husband	• Call to say I'm thinking about her • Make the bed when I get up because I know she likes it made	• Remembering • Time	• Post-it note on computer at work • Set alarm for 3 minutes earlier
Living a healthy life to see my grandchildren grow up	• Eat three servings of vegetables a day • Limit red meat to one time per week	• Not having good vegetables on hand • Fast-food lunch at work	• Shopping on weekend to stock up • Pack lunch evening before

You should experiment and see what would work best for you. Our only suggestion is to make sure that the list is written down and is placed somewhere you'll see it every day. We should give one note of caution about the format above: The man who created the format and list above posted *all* of his values on his refrigerator. The first time he called his wife at work to say he was thinking about her, she asked him why he hadn't made the bed that morning! Thus, if you have goals related to family members (who also might use the refrigerator) that you don't want them to see, they might be better listed somewhere that you alone will see them every day.

Summing It Up

Values provide a compass for determining the direction of a meaningful life, and goals related to those values provide destinations along the way.

Remember that barriers such as time constraints, limited energy, and negative feelings or thoughts will come up, but that these do not change the direction you want to be heading.

PART II

Diabetes Acceptance

CHAPTER 4

What Have You Tried?

U nless you found out this morning that you were diagnosed with diabetes, chances are you have tried plenty of things in order to manage and cope with it. The strategies you have tried, both successful and unsuccessful, are the focus of this chapter. We will determine what your most common strategies are and examine what has worked and what hasn't in your efforts to deal with your general thoughts and feelings and those about having diabetes.

Diabetes? Who Me?

For many people, disbelief is the first reaction to receiving a diabetes diagnosis. Disbelief, or even outright denial, can often be a stage of coping that occurs as part of the process of adjusting to a permanent problem. For example, it can be one stage along the way to anger, sadness, and eventually acceptance. However, some people really never come out of the disbelief phase; the news that they have diabetes and need to make all of these changes to their lifestyle is just too painful and overwhelming. People have many ways to push difficult thoughts and feelings to the side. Disbelief, in this sense, is a way to have life go on in the way it was before without having to deal with too many changes.

For instance, take the example of Tom, a fifty-five-year-old contractor who has worked his entire life in construction only to develop a back injury in his fifties that made him have to stop working. Not working and having a back injury would reasonably lead anybody to become less active and put on extra weight, both of which happened to Tom. Months later he noticed that he was feeling thirsty all the time, even though he wasn't going outside or exercising, and at his next checkup for his back, he mentioned this to his doctor. His doctor ordered a test for diabetes, and the results came back positive. For Tom, the news was unbelievable. His perception of himself and his life had changed so much in such a short time: from an active, working man who was busy every day building things to an injured man with diabetes who stayed home all day. This was just too much for Tom to face head-on. He decided that the test must have been an error and went home and went about his life without telling anybody, including his wife, about the test.

What Are the Costs?

This process is understandable, and it even seems to have some benefits. For instance, by pushing away difficult thoughts about having diabetes, it might seem as though the stress about having diabetes is reduced. While this might be true in the short term, it's not true in the long term; there could potentially be some real costs to you if you deny your diabetes for too long.

First of all, there may be real costs to your health. If you're not willing to admit that you have diabetes or are trying hard not to think about it very often, it is very difficult to do all of the many things you need to do every day to take care of your diabetes, things like eating well, exercising, taking your medication, and testing your blood sugar. As anybody with diabetes knows, these things are hard enough to accomplish if you are completely aware of and focused on your diabetes. Adding in disbelief about your diabetes diagnosis and its meaning only makes things harder! Ironically, denying your diabetes and not taking care of yourself to ensure that you don't have to think about your diabetes also can affect your stress levels negatively.

This result may seem counterintuitive, because it's the opposite of what many people intend when they try to avoid focusing on their diabetes or reject the idea that they have it. However, not taking care of your diabetes can lead to diabetic reactions and complications that can definitely add stress to your life long-term. Below is an example of how this cycle operates.

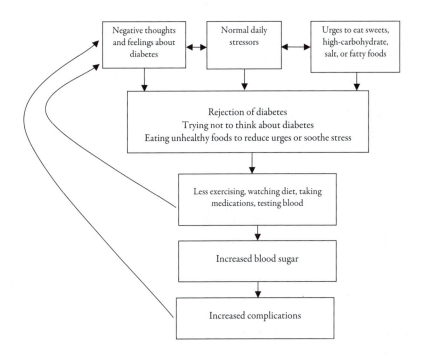

Negative thoughts and feelings about having diabetes, urges to eat unhealthy foods or not exercise, and normal daily stresses all can lead a person with diabetes to reject or deny their diabetes or to try not to think about it. But this leads to less of the things necessary to take care of diabetes, which we know leads to higher blood sugar.

The other problem is that deep down, avoidance cannot work, because it's not possible to trick ourselves into thinking something we don't really think, to feeling something we don't really feel, or to not knowing something that we really do know. This process can increase a person's stress and add guilt or frustration to the negative experiences they are having. Over time, when higher blood sugar leads to more complications like cardiovascular problems, nerve pain, sexual dysfunction, and the like, even more efforts must be made to keep not thinking about or denying diabetes, as well as the new fears and worries that are related to it. These conditions are much more likely to increase stress rather than decrease it.

The story of Tom from above is a good example of this pattern. A year or so after his diagnosis he began noticing a tingling in his feet that became very painful at night when he was trying to sleep. He went to see his doctor, who informed him that he had developed the beginning stages of nerve damage in his feet, which had been caused by long-term out-of-control blood sugar values. Although his doctor prescribed a medication that lessened the tingling and pain in his feet, the damage Tom had done was never completely reversible. What had begun as a way to deal with his stress by trying not to think of himself as a person with diabetes had increased his stress overall in the longterm.

Common Ways of Avoiding Diabetes Thoughts and Feelings

Out-and-out denial as in Tom's case is not likely among readers of this book. The very fact that you are reading it indicates that you're taking another, healthier path. But there are subtler ways to push away fears. We all have strategies and things we say to ourselves in order to avoid dealing with difficult experiences. Below are some frequent things we hear from people with diabetes.

"My Diabetes Isn't Really That Big of a Deal"

This is one of the most common statements we hear from people with diabetes. One of the first things that people diagnosed with diabetes often try to do is to keep their life as normal as possible. It's hard to keep believing that your life hasn't changed, however, when you are placed on an unending diet and are told to spend your leisure time poking yourself, checking your body for complications, and engaging in appropriate exercise. The result of this contradiction is that patients minimize what their diabetes really means. In fact, we have met patients who have successfully kept themselves from fully understanding that they have diabetes for decades. Not surprisingly, these people never really have control of their diabetes. In fact, we would say their diabetes always has control of them.

"It's Only a Small Piece of Chocolate Cake"

Denying the effects of not managing diabetes is tempting. Denying the power one has to control this disease is even more tempting. The strategy of not educating yourself about what you should and shouldn't eat and what you need to do to manage your diabetes is one way that you might try to avoid dealing with your feelings about your illness. Take the case of Joe, a thirty-eight-year-old man with diabetes who came into our clinic weighing 375 pounds. He told us that he was in excruciating pain due to his diabetes and recently had needed to go onto disability from his job as an office manager because he was unable to sit at his desk all day and during his forty-five-minute commute to work. Although he had had diabetes for four years at the time, Joe reported that he had no idea what was recommended for him in terms of his diet. When we explored things further, we found that he was eating nearly the opposite of a diabetes diet, and that his food intake was completely tied to his mood and his cravings for comfort food. In essence, Joe's way of not dealing with his feelings about his diabetes was not to deny that he had diabetes or that it was a big deal, but to keep himself completely in the dark about what diabetes management would mean.

"My Vision Isn't Really All That Different"

Many people experience small changes in their body as a result of their diabetes. Often these changes do not represent the severe complications the person is worried about. For example, vision changes, including blurriness and focusing problems, are common when a person is first diagnosed with diabetes and result from the out-of-control blood sugars that often occur before the person and their physician realize that diabetes is present. These vision changes do not typically represent the long-term vision loss that can sometimes occur as a complication of diabetes, but changes in vision make many people with diabetes concerned that vision loss is imminent. Many times, rather than deal with the immediate experience and take steps to correct the problem, patients become worried about the possibilities it represents and attempt to avoid thinking about these body changes in order to protect themselves from the worry of what it could be.

"It's Unfair That Other People Can Eat Whatever They Want and I Can't"

One thing is for sure: having diabetes is unfair. Many of our patients over the years have started their first interaction with their doctor, nutritionist, or behavioral therapist with this sentence. We are quick to agree on this one. It is absolutely unfair. However, the strategy of focusing on the fact that it is unfair when others eat foods that are high in sugar and fat and you can't is one way to *not* deal with your diabetes-related feelings.

One example of this type of avoidance was experienced by a woman who came to our clinic for help coping with her diabetes. Her name was Lois, and she was a sixty-eight-year-old former nurse who led a very active life in her retirement. She had recently been diagnosed with diabetes, and had been trying to make the lifestyle changes recommended by her doctor. But she found that she was having an impossible time because none of her friends had diabetes, so all of her social engagements involved food that she was supposed to keep out of her diet. She told us that she didn't think it was fair that she couldn't eat the pastries and cakes that were always present at her social gatherings, and because of this she rarely passed these treats up. Over time, we learned that Lois's focus on the fairness of the situation, however accurate, was her way to feel in control of her situation and prevented her from feeling all the fear and isolation she had felt since being diagnosed.

"I Don't Need to Take My Medication, I Feel Fine"

This is a classic statement made by many people with diabetes. The fact that diabetes is present even when you experience no symptoms makes this one of the toughest diseases to treat. The approach of not managing diabetes when symptoms are not present is often related to trying to let oneself believe that diabetes is somehow temporary, or that it might have gone away or improved over time because there are no symptoms present. The most important thing to remember about diabetes is that the symptoms do not need to be present for complications to be developing or present. Many people experience changes "all of a sudden" or "out of the blue" when they think that things are going along well. However, the only way to really know if things are going well is to check your blood sugar often, to get your HbA$_{1C}$ checked regularly, and to continue to take any medication and make lifestyle changes prescribed (see chapter 9 for developing your own plan to do this). While it might be tempting to believe that if symptoms are not present then your diabetes has somehow gone away, this is just another strategy for avoiding the negative feelings, in this case by trying to replace them with more positive ones.

"I Refuse to Be One of Those Diabetes Food-Freaks"

We have had many patients say that the sacrifices required in the management of diabetes are too much, particularly the sacrifices people feel they need to make regarding food. One patient, Kirk, a forty-seven-year-old married man with two small children, told his doctor that he didn't think that a life full of sacrifice is worth living. He stated that he would rather have a shorter life than spend the rest of his time watching every piece of food he put into his mouth. Kirk, like many people with diabetes, uses this all-or-nothing strategy to avoid the difficult work of managing his diabetes and his feelings about it. It is much more difficult to admit that there are many stages between not caring for one's diabetes and spending all of one's time and energy on their diabetes.

The Super Strategy: Push Away Your Feelings and Thoughts

If you look closely you may be able to see that all of these strategies have a common element. They are all ways that people try to push away the difficult feelings and thoughts that come up when they are diagnosed with diabetes. Unfortunately, having difficult feelings and thoughts is part of the process of dealing with a chronic disease. Pushing away difficult feelings and thoughts is kind of like trying to throw flypaper: the more we try to disengage from it, the more tangled up we get.

How Do *You* Cope with Having Diabetes?

We all have strategies for dealing with difficult things, whether they are out-and-out denial or methods like taking a walk or talking with a friend. Some of these strategies make coping with the hard things we encounter in our life easier, and some of them make these hard things more complicated. In the case of Tom, the construction worker with the back injury, his strategy of rejecting his diagnosis was designed to make the situation less stressful for him, and in the end it not only made things more complicated but also more stressful.

In order to determine your strategies for coping with painful or hard situations, think back to situations in your life where you have really struggled. Maybe it was when you found out you had diabetes, or maybe it was a time you experienced a painful breakup or lost somebody or something that was close to you. What types of things did you do to deal with the situation? Did you spend more time in bed or withdraw from friends and family? Did you seek the support of others or social activities to get your mind off things? Did you turn to drugs, alcohol, or other methods to help numb your feelings? Did you seek professional help from a therapist or doctor? Did you throw yourself into your work and take on extra tasks to fill the time so you wouldn't have to sit around and think about things? Or maybe you did many of these things at the same time or for different stressors. Take out your diabetes journal and list two or three strategies that are common for you or that you notice you did when you think about a time that you have struggled in the past. These are important to keep track of, because they are likely to be strategies you will use in dealing with thoughts and feelings related to this challenge as well.

Person in the Hole

Now that you have your coping strategies in mind, let's try a little imagination exercise. This exercise is from Steve Hayes, Kirk Strosahl, and Kelly Wilson's 1999 book on acceptance and commitment therapy, and it will provide us with a way to see how automatic your strategies for dealing with your worries and reactions to having diabetes are, as well as a way to determine how they are working for you.

First, imagine that you are taken up for a ride in a helicopter. While you're in the helicopter, imagine that you are blindfolded and given a tool bag. At some point, the helicopter touches down to the ground, and you are told that your job in life is to run around in the field you have been dropped off in. What you don't know (and can't see because you are blindfolded) is that there are a number of widely spaced, very large holes throughout the field. So you run around in the field for a while, running up hills and around in circles, and eventually you fall into one of the holes. Finding that you are stuck, you take off your blindfold and reach into the tool bag, figuring that it must contain some way out of this hole, since the people who dropped you off here gave you the bag. When you reach into the bag, however, you find only a shovel. So you dig a little bit here and a little bit there, and after a while you notice that instead of being out of the hole, you are only further down in it. Now the question is: what would you do to get out of this hole? Think about it for a minute and write down the first thing that you think you would do in this situation to try to solve it.

What did you come up with? Whatever response you came up with, think about times you have been "stuck in a hole" in your life before. Did you come up with a very similar type of solution then as well? For example, if you came up with a logical solution to being stuck in this hole, such as digging stairs or a ramp to get out, did you also notice that you came up with logical solutions to other "holes" in your life, such as trying to figure the problem out analytically or logically? For example, maybe after finding out you had diabetes, you read everything you could get your hands on in order to "figure it out" and reduce your worry about it. If so, maybe trying to approach situations that worry you or cause anxiety or stress with logic is your main strategy for coping with them.

Another solution that people often come up with to this dilemma is that they would shout for help. If you came up with this solution, think about your life for a moment. Does this sound like you? Are you somebody who often tries to cope with stress by getting others' help and talking about it with friends and family? If so, then calling for help may be the coping strategy that we need to pay attention to when stressors arise in coping with your diabetes.

What else have you come up with? Maybe you decided right away that since the shovel wasn't working, then maybe there is no solution, and you decided that you would just do what you could to make the hole comfortable and resign yourself to staying in it. If so, does this sound like something you would do in other situations? Is it like you to give in to the situation and try to make the best of it? If so, again, this may be the strategy we need to keep an eye on as difficult thoughts and feelings about your diabetes come up.

What else comes to mind? Maybe you keep coming up with solutions that are similar in theme. For example, Paul, a fifty-seven-year-old man recently diagnosed with type 2 diabetes, was having a difficult time managing his blood sugar. He came to see us because he couldn't seem to get himself motivated to take care of his diabetes. When Paul did this exercise, he first suggested that he would dig stairs in the dirt with his shovel. We pointed out that this was a very logical solution, and he agreed that he tended to solve most problems in his life with logic. When we asked him what else he would try, if digging stairs did not work, he said that he would dig a ramp in the dirt with his shovel. When asked what he would try if that also did not work, he stated that he would use the shovel as a lever to catapult himself out of the hole. As we talked more with him about his feelings about having diabetes, he told us that he didn't think it was logical for him to dwell on his worries about his diabetes, and so he tried not to think about them. Unfortunately for Paul, not "dwelling" on them meant that he ended up not thinking about his diabetes—and thus not managing it well. When we asked him to list the areas where logic was working for him and where it wasn't, he quickly identified that while logic worked well in many areas of his life, it wasn't working in his dealing with his worry and anxiety about having diabetes, and it was preventing him from managing his diabetes effectively. He reported that using logic in those situations was just like using the shovel to try to get out of a hole—that the more he used this tool that seemed as though it would work, the further down he seemed to find himself.

So why did we have you do this exercise? First, we wanted to help shed some light on what your particular strategies for dealing with tough situations are. Are you a person who tries to solve them logically, like the patient above? Or are you more likely to go to others for support? Or maybe you're somebody who resigns themselves to the situation. Whatever your most handy strategies are, it is useful to be aware of them.

Once you know what your commons strategies are, the second thing this exercise is designed to do is to help you evaluate where they are useful and where they aren't. For instance, while logic, calling for help, or resigning oneself to a situation all might work in some situations, there may be other situations where they are not useful. Often, the places where these strategies do not work as well are situations where they are used to try to push down or avoid difficult emotions. Keep in mind that this does not mean that these strategies don't work in many situations, including in many areas of managing your diabetes. They just may not help much with managing your *feelings* and *thoughts* about your diabetes in every situation. Since keeping difficult thoughts and feelings at bay is the "super strategy" underlying all forms of avoidance, even otherwise very effective problem-solving approaches can be ineffective here. While these strategies might help in the short term, they may not be that effective in the long term if they are used to push away the real feelings going on.

But I Like My Strategies!

Examining the usefulness of your strategies for dealing with difficult emotions, whether you are struggling with anxiety, depression, diabetes, the loss of a loved one, or just day-to-day stress, may make you feel that these strategies, although they may not be perfect, are all you've got. This may make you feel uncomfortable with the idea of giving them up or trying something new. The purpose of this investigation, however, is not to change things in areas that are working well, but rather to give you some new options in the areas that are not working well. For instance, in the case of Paul, the patient with the logical solutions, we weren't interested in changing the many areas of his life where logic was useful—including the areas of diabetes management where being logical was effective (such as his logical approach to learning about dietary changes and their effect on his blood sugar, which he learned by testing in a methodical manner). Rather, our interest in targeting his logical strategies was confined to dealing with his emotions this way, since it meant he was trying so hard to control his thoughts and feelings that it was getting in the way of his taking care of his diabetes.

Quicksand

Another way to think about the issue of trying to control feelings is to think about quicksand (Hayes, Strosahl, and Wilson 1999). When you are in quicksand, what is the first thing you want to do? For most of us, the answer is to struggle to get out as fast as we can. But is that the best strategy for getting out of quicksand? Not at all. When you want to get out of quicksand, the best strategy is to lie down as flat as possible, distributing your weight evenly across the quicksand. From there, you can inch across to safety; but it is very important to put as much of your body in contact with the quicksand as possible. This generally feels like the exact opposite of what you should do, but unlike the strategy of trying to stand up or run to safety, this is the strategy that works.

It is often the same with difficult thoughts and feelings. The strategy that feels the most appropriate is to get the heck away from them, and this is often the first tool we pull out when we are dealing with painful thoughts and feelings. Often, though, the strategy that works the best for dealing with emotions is to do the exact opposite of our tried-and-true strategies and lean into these feelings. While it may feel as though the best thing to do is to move *away* from bad feelings, sometimes the most effective thing to do is to move *toward* your values, even if that means coming in more contact with bad feelings.

A Note of Caution

It may be tempting, as you read this, to start forming rules for yourself about what is the best strategy to use when difficult feelings come up for you related to your diabetes or your life in general. You may think back on the example of the person in the hole, or the quicksand, and think to yourself that any time you try to avoid or control your feelings, you are failing in your attempts to deal with them, or that you are "doing it wrong." It is important that we make it clear here that the purpose of this discussion is to help you understand where you potentially *are* able to make changes and where you likely *aren't*. You can change the strategies you use for dealing with difficult thoughts or feelings. You just cannot easily change what these thoughts or feelings are.

You will still be pulled to try to change or control your thoughts and feelings, and chances are you will continue to engage in strategies to try to avoid or deny them from time to time. This is just human nature. We aren't saying that these strategies never work or that to have a full life you should never engage them. Rather, we want to help you notice when they work and when they don't, so that your own experience can guide you in what will work best in a given situation. To do that we have to go beyond the normal avoidant super strategy. In the chapters ahead, we will lay out a new way of approaching your stress, worry, or other feelings and thoughts you may want to try to control or eliminate, and we will give you the opportunity to try out these new strategies so that you can be as effective as possible in moving toward your values and goals.

Summing It Up

Trying to change or control your thoughts and feelings may not work in the long term and may cost you in your ability to take care of your diabetes.

While you may not have control over automatic feelings or thoughts, you do have control over the strategies you use to deal with them.

CHAPTER 5

Who Are You?

A crucial element for understanding how to relate to our thoughts and feelings about having diabetes is to understand what the relationship is between our thoughts, our feelings, and our selves. What we mean by this is that before we can determine a good strategy for managing thoughts and feelings about diabetes, we have to have an understanding that there is a difference between what we think and feel and the person doing the thinking and feeling.

To begin with, it helps to spend a little time talking about what we mean when we use the word "self." The word self in this instance refers to the person who is doing the thinking and feeling. When we say "myself" or "yourself," we are actually not talking about all the thoughts and feelings I or you have, but of the person who is thinking or feeling.

Conceptualized Self

There is one aspect of each of us that is very important: the way we see ourselves. The way we see ourselves, or as Hayes, Strosahl, and Wilson (1999) describe it, our *conceptualized self*, gives us lots of information about what type of picture we carry around of ourselves. Maybe we think of ourselves as "the nice one" or "the organized one," or maybe we carry around some old labels of ourselves from childhood, such as "the stupid one" or "the quiet one." Whatever the label, whether positive or negative, the way we conceptualize ourselves plays a very big role in how we live our lives.

For instance, take the example of Joanna, a fifty-six-year-old mother of two grown children. Throughout her life, Joanna has made sacrifices for her husband and children. Because she had children early in her life, she put off going to college to become a teacher, a dream she had had since she was a little girl. Instead, she took part-time office jobs to help put her husband through school to become an art historian. These jobs allowed her to be home for her children after school and to have a nice home for her family.

When Joanna was asked how she defines herself, she said that she is always "the helpful one." She said that whenever a friend or family member needed anything, she would always drop what she was doing and go and help out. She said that part of how she thought of herself was as the person whose needs and wants could always be put aside to make room for the needs and wants of her family, since she saw it as her job to sacrifice whatever was necessary to take care of them in any way she could. It is important to note that Joanna was very proud to describe herself this way; being somebody that everybody could count on was a very big value for her, and she felt as though making sacrifices for others was part of what made her a good person.

When Joanna came into our clinic in order to get help in dealing with her diabetes, one thing became clear very quickly: because Joanna had conceptualized herself as somebody who always made sacrifices for others, it was nearly impossible for her to spend the time, energy, and focus needed to manage her diabetes, particularly if it meant taking time and focus away from her family. When asked what she thought the difficulty was for her in creating time and focus to manage her diabetes, Joanna told us, "I'm not the kind of person who focuses on myself. I'm a giver."

Conceptualizing herself as a "giver" was very important for Joanna, and it allowed her to think of herself in a way that was positive for her. The problem, however, was that this conceptualization had hardened into stone; Joanna felt as though she was unable to change her behavior because of her conceptualization of herself. Even when it meant not being able to take care of her diabetes, something that was very important for Joanna, her role as a giver felt too powerful to change.

Self-Awareness

In order for Joanna to understand the role of her conceptualized self, it was important that she pay attention to her thoughts, feelings, and values and spend some time sorting out the differences between them. This step requires *self-awareness*—noticing what thoughts, feelings, bodily sensations, memories, and experiences you are having. The trick here is the ability to be aware of your thoughts and feelings while not being sucked into their being true. For example, consider Joanna's experiences again. She probably had a number of thoughts and feelings that contributed to her understanding of herself as a giver. She may have had positive feelings of being useful or important when her family relied on her. She may have had some negative feelings or thoughts about being useless or meaningless when her family didn't need her in order to make it through the day. She may have felt some loneliness or some unhappy feelings or thoughts about the choices she made in those times. She may have felt regret for not making choices related to what she wanted in her life, or she may have felt satisfaction and pleasure when remembering her life with small children and the amazing experience of being able to be there to raise them.

Perhaps when Joanna thinks about her life currently, she experiences a range of happy and sad emotions. Maybe she feels lost about what to do now that her children are older. She could feel disconnected from her husband, given the differences in their lives now that their children are not the daily thread that they once were. Or she may feel a sense of freedom and openness to new possibilities and a renewed connection to her husband now that they have time to focus on their relationship without the demands of child rearing.

Whatever Joanna is feeling, the second component of understanding what we are is in understanding what we are experiencing in this moment, here, today. Knowing what we are feeling in the moment is a difficult task by any account, and if Joanna is less than familiar with her daily experiences, nobody could blame her. Most of us go days or weeks without really examining what we are feeling or experiencing in the moment. We sometimes talk about this as being "on autopilot" and just cruising through our lives.

Why would this autopiloting occur? One reason might be that many of the things we have to experience during a given day are difficult or challenging to manage. For instance, if we have a hard day, there can be numerous negative thoughts, feelings, or experiences that all heap on us at once, and it is easier to check out than to try to deal with them simultaneously. If this experience occurs frequently enough, it becomes more and more difficult to be present in the moment, because we get used to being on autopilot, and this state is often more comfortable than dealing with difficult thoughts and feelings all the time. However, this checking out prevents us, like Joanna, from having a sense of our real feelings, and we may not only miss large portions of our lives, but we may also rely on our conceptualized self to understand our experience, rather than actually being aware of what we think and feel.

One way to increase our ability to notice what is happening is to train ourselves to do the noticing. This skill is a little like lifting weights to build up a muscle; it isn't very difficult to do, but it takes consistent practice to see results over time. You can start with the exercise below to see how much you can notice about the present, and continue to practice it and other exercises described in this book to build up this awareness muscle.

Overpass Exercise

This exercise is designed to help you become more aware and mindful of what you are thinking and feeling right now, in this moment. First, read the whole exercise through, and then try it out with your eyes closed. It's okay if you don't remember all of the components of what is written; the purpose of the exercise is to notice your experience in the moment, so try to not get too hung up on whether or not you are doing it correctly. Just pay attention to the moment.

First, close your eyes and notice what you hear, feel, smell, and sense in the place where you are. Pay attention to what the air feels like on your skin, and what your body feels like in the position you're in. Next, imagine a freeway overpass with cars driving past in both directions. It doesn't matter if the overpass is one that you know of or one that you come up with in your imagination. Now picture yourself sitting underneath this overpass in such a way that you can still see the cars going by, but they are over your head. Next, imagine that you can take individual thoughts from your mind and place them gently on the cars driving by overhead. Imagine that you can observe each of your thoughts sitting on top of a car, without attempting to stop them or evaluate them, but just noticing them. You may have to slow the cars down some to get your thoughts onto them and to be able to watch them as they drive away.

Notice what thoughts you have right now, and select one. Now try placing it on a car on the overpass in your mind's eye. It's okay if you have a hard time finding a thought to place on the car; it might take a little while to get the hang of this. If you have the thought that you can't find a thought to place on the car, try placing *that* thought (that you can't find a thought) on a car. Or, if you are thinking that you are not doing this exercise right or catching on fast enough, try placing that thought (that you are doing this incorrectly) on a car. If the process feels silly or you have a hard time keeping the thought on a car, try placing that thought (that this process feels silly or that you're having a hard time) on a car.

Once you have a thought on a car, see if you can just notice the thought as it drives by on the bridge. If you notice evaluations or other thoughts popping up in response to the thought on the car, see if you can place those thoughts onto cars and observe them driving by as well. Notice if you find yourself getting stuck to a thought, or climbing up onto the car to try to stay with the thought. Notice if you find yourself trying to throw a thought onto a car to separate it from yourself. If you lose track of the exercise, back up a few moments and try to see what happened right before you lost it. Continue noticing your thoughts and placing them on cars for about five minutes, and then you can open your eyes back up.

So, how did you do? Were you able to place the thoughts onto the cars? Again, it's okay if you weren't able to do it this time, or if you had to read a little, practice a little, and read some more. Continue practicing and see if you can do it next time. The most important thing is not really being able to put all the thoughts on the cars, but beginning to observe your thoughts more freely and to notice how the thoughts on the cars are different from the person noticing them.

This exercise also contains another lesson: certain thoughts are harder to let drive by. The ones that knock you off of the overpass are ones we will begin to learn how to deal with in new ways.

Noticing Self

So who is this "self"? You might think about your self as made up of your conceptualized self, combined with the self-awareness of the experiences and thoughts from the exercise above. There is one more aspect of the self, which we will call the *noticing self* (the "observer self" in Hayes, Strosahl, and Wilson 1999). The noticing self is "the you behind the you." Ordinarily, we think about our self, if we think about it at all, as made up of some combination of our history, our thoughts and feelings, our roles, and our physical body. However, for our purposes, the noticing self is an important and useful way to think about who we are.

Noticing-Self Exercise

To get a better sense of this, it is helpful to do another little exercise (adapted from Hayes, Strosahl, and Wilson 1999). Right now (as soon as you finish reading this paragraph), close your eyes and no matter where you are, pay attention to where you are and what you are doing. Notice the sounds around you, the feeling of the air on your skin, any scents, or other sensations available. Notice any thoughts, feelings, and memories that come into your awareness as well, and do this for about thirty seconds. Then continue reading.

Welcome back. What did you notice? Were you aware of the sounds, fragrances, sensations, thoughts, feelings, and memories that were present for you? Were you able to notice what was going on around you? Good. Next, notice who it was that was noticing those things.

Now think back on a memory from last year. It doesn't matter if it is a good memory or a bad memory, or if it feels important or insignificant. Use whatever memory that pops into your head. When you've found a memory (and after you finish reading this paragraph), close your eyes again, and imagine climbing inside that memory and noticing all the same things you did here in the present a minute ago. Notice what you hear from within that memory, notice what is going on around you, and what the air feels like on your skin. Sense any odors, or people, or sensations present. Note the thoughts, feelings, bodily sensations, or memories that you were having. The more you can notice from "within your skin" from that experience, the better (Hayes, Strosahl, and Wilson 1999).

Next pick a memory from when you were a teenager. Again, it doesn't matter if the memory is good or bad, big or little. Insert yourself into this memory as well, and again notice what you hear, feel, think, smell, and notice from inside that memory. Do any sensations or emotions stand out? Notice what you are doing and who you are with, as well as the sights and sounds around you.

So what did you notice *across* these three experiences? And, more importantly, who was doing the noticing? The person who was noticing the sounds and sensations in the place you are in today, right now, as you read this was in some important sense the same person noticing the sounds and sensations earlier in your life, or you would not know these things happened to "you." Did the experiences and thoughts and feelings you noticed change over time? Were there similarities? If so, can you tell that the person who was noticing those similarities and differences is somebody who is separate from those experiences, thoughts, and feelings?

This is kind of a tricky idea, so it's okay if it feels a little confusing at first. Basically, for each of these situations (the moment as you were noticing things a few minutes ago, the memory from last year, and the memory from when you were a teenager), there were all kinds of things to notice: sounds, scents, feelings, thoughts, sensations—and then there was somebody there who was noticing those things. We call that somebody the noticing self because this is the part of you who stays consistent across time to notice these things occurring.

What Makes Up My Noticing Self?

Many times patients tell us that they are made up of all of their experiences, and that it is these experiences that define who they are. While this is true in some sense, it's useful to think about there being a separate *you* that is distinct from all of your experiences. This is because, if your noticing self has been around to notice all of your life experiences, it doesn't quite make sense that the you that was noticing them is the same you that is made up of them. Confused? It might be clearer to talk about each of the things it seems our "selves" are made up of one by one.

Maybe my noticing self is made up of my history or past experiences. First off, think about your history or past experiences. Are these you? Try to imagine all of your memories loaded into a computer. Would that be all of you? Probably not. For most of us, the experiences we have had in the past feel very important, but they aren't the self that was just noticing the sounds, scents, and feeling of the air in the exercise in the previous section.

Maybe my noticing self is made up of my thoughts and feelings. Another way we often think about our selves is as a combination of all of our thoughts and feelings. A patient once put this belief perfectly when he said, "Of course I'm my thoughts—who else would I be?" Other patients assert that even if they aren't completely made up of their thoughts, feelings, and experiences that these have at least dramatically changed who they are over the years. A great example of this was given by a patient who had experienced really traumatic war zone experiences in early adulthood. He stated that he was now a completely different person than he had been before he went to war. What he eventually realized, however, was that while his past experiences were important to his present experiences and choices, there was somebody there who noticed his thoughts, feelings, and experiences before the war and who could compare them to the thoughts, feelings, and experiences after the war. If he was a completely different person based on these different experiences, he would not have the ability to compare the two.

Maybe my noticing self is made up of my roles. You may feel that "you" are a combination of your roles. For instance, people will often say "I am a mother" or "I am an attorney" when asked to describe themselves. Think for a moment about the roles you play throughout the day. You might be a commuter, a customer, an employee, a boss, a parker, a shopper, or a mom, dad, brother, sister, daughter, son, grandmother, grandfather, or cousin, just to name a few. While it may seem as though these roles are what you're made of, one thing to notice is that there is somebody there who takes on all these roles who is consistent throughout the days, weeks, months, and years. In other words, while your roles may change dramatically over time, there is somebody who takes on each of the roles who does not change. That somebody is the noticing self.

Maybe my noticing self is made up of my body. Finally, we often think of our selves as our physical body. Nothing else feels quite as solid an indication of who we are as the body we inhabit; a notion that is accentuated by the fact that when our bodies fail, we stop living. Actually, the body that you have today is probably made up of a completely different set of cells than the body that you had when you were very young, given that the cells in our bodies only live for a limited amount of time before they are replaced by new cells. And if you think about the body you had when you were a small child, there probably isn't much of a resemblance to the body that is reading this book right now. There may be facial features or a body shape that is similar, but the differences between the two bodies probably far outweigh the similarities.

If you think about the transformation of your body over time— from the time you were a young child barely able to see over a table, to an adolescent awkwardly coming into the body of an adult, to an adult possibly watching the effects of time change the body yet again—you notice that there is a person observing these changes over time. This person remains consistent from year to year, even as the body changes, and can think back on the body of years ago and compare it to the present version. This, again, is the noticing self.

So, while our history, our roles, our bodies, and our thoughts, feelings, and experiences can feel as though they are the self that defines us, they all have variation and changes over time that are observed by somebody. For our purposes, it is that somebody that we consider you—your noticing self.

Chessboard Exercise

There is a very good reason why we are talking about your noticing self in order to help you manage your diabetes. It is to help create a space where any of the scary thoughts and feelings about having diabetes is okay to have, while still taking care of yourself and your diabetes. One core way of thinking about this from an ACT perspective is what is called the Chessboard Exercise (Hayes, Strosahl, and Wilson 1999).

First, imagine that you have a chessboard in front of you that is enormous. Imagine that it goes infinitely in all directions. Now imagine that on this chessboard, there are the usual pieces you would find in a chess game: kings, queens, rooks, knights, bishops, and pawns. It's okay if you don't know how to play chess or you don't know very much about the game; most of us can imagine what a chessboard looks like without too much knowledge of chess itself. Imagine that half of the chess pieces are red and half of them are white. The red pieces in our game are made up of thoughts and feelings that you don't like: maybe things like negative thoughts or feelings, or fears about losing your eyesight or your feet to diabetes. The white pieces in our game are made up of the positive thoughts and feelings you could have: maybe happiness at a good meter reading, or optimistic thoughts about getting control of your diabetes.

So in our game of chess, we have essentially five separate entities. We have the white pieces, the red pieces, the player for the red team, the player for the white team, and the board. If we imagine that this game of chess is you, which of these entities would you say you are? For example, are you the white player, trying to move the white pieces (positive thoughts and feelings about your diabetes) into a position to win and remove all of the red pieces (negative thoughts and feelings about your diabetes)? Or are you the white pieces themselves, fighting against negative thoughts and feelings about diabetes? Maybe some days you feel as though you are the red pieces or player—knocking off any positive thoughts or feelings and just focused on the negative ones. Or maybe you are the board, the place where all of the action happens.

Most of us spend the majority of our time being either the white player or the white pieces. We are fighting against the red pieces, trying to knock them off the board and get rid of them once and for all. This is the most commonsense approach to take with negative thoughts and feelings; get rid of them and increase the positive thoughts and feelings. But remember what we said about the board: that it is enormous and goes infinitely in all directions. Thus, it is not possible to completely knock these pieces off the board. This is consistent with what we talked about in chapter 1: no matter how hard you try not to think about a purple dragon, your anxiety, or even your diabetes, it generally does not go away just because you want it to.

So what about being the board instead of the white player or white pieces? If you are the board, you no longer care as much about the outcome of the game, so you no longer need to fight to try to get rid of particular pieces. In addition, as the board you are not in danger if a really big piece comes along, like anxiety or sadness. It cannot threaten you in the same way as it would if you were a chess piece coming up against it in a fight. Thus, not only do you have less need to eliminate negative thoughts and feelings, but your perspective of how dangerous they are changes as well.

So What Do Boards Do?

What can this board do, then, if it can't be used as a launching pad for pieces that we don't want or are tired of dealing with? Well, in this metaphor, there are two things that your board can do: it can hold pieces (both good and bad), and it can move in a direction carrying them all. Now actually, since we said that the board goes infinitely in all directions, it technically can't move anywhere that it isn't already covering, but we'll pretend that the giant board can move around anyway.

So, if the two things this board can do are hold pieces and move in a direction, what does that mean in terms of you and your life with diabetes? Well, you, as the board, can now have your positive thoughts about your diabetes, like those that say you will be able to manage your blood sugar and stay on track. And you can also have your negative thoughts, like your worry about losing your battle with diabetes or thoughts that you can't make all of these difficult changes in your life. And the reason you can have *both* of these kinds of thoughts is that, as the board, you don't need to get rid of them in order to move forward.

And where can you go if you are able to move forward? In the direction of your values, of course. This means that you can move toward close relationships, or taking care of your diabetes, or living an active life, while holding on to the thoughts and feelings that feel as though they could stop you. You can literally bring them along with you for the ride.

Louis's Story

For a clearer example of how this works, take the case of Louis, a fifty-seven-year-old man diagnosed with type 2 diabetes. He spent the first year after his diagnosis in a deep depression, because he felt as though he would never again be able to do all of the things that he enjoyed. He worried constantly about his blood sugar and his ever-rising blood pressure and cholesterol, but he felt completely powerless to change his eating and exercise habits and often didn't feel like taking his medication because of the way it made him feel.

When we first started talking about the idea of the chessboard, Louis said that it didn't feel as though it applied to him. He was doing the best he could and really didn't feel as though it was his thoughts and feelings as much as his situation that was standing in his way. We talked him into trying it out anyway, and he found he was able to identify many positive white pieces/thoughts, including his hope that he would find some willpower soon and his belief that he was a good person and that good people were not punished with terrible outcomes if they did not deserve them. He also found that he was able to find many negative red pieces/thoughts that he was using these white pieces to fight against. These included all of his thoughts and worries about what could happen to him and his not feeling like taking care of his diabetes or taking his medication.

Louis quickly realized that he was living his life within the struggle between these two types of pieces. He stated that he was always trying to fight against his worries or make them go away by trying to kick them off the board and not think about them. He noticed that he was trying to change the way he felt about taking his medication by trying to convince himself that it wasn't really that bad. Interestingly, he also observed that one of the pieces he was struggling the most with was his strong desire for sweets after dinner. He told us that he had tried every strategy he could think of to make these urges for sweets go away, and that he usually ended up giving in to them. He said that he felt as though he was in a life-or-death war with these urges, and that they were winning because they were so much stronger than his willpower.

One key aspect of Louis's experience was his realization that he was fighting at "piece level" rather than at "board level." When he switched his perspective, he found that he did not need to eliminate the urges, but that he could notice them and see them for what they were: urges. From this space, Louis had an opportunity to do something different with regard to eating sweets after dinner. In other words, he was able to move *toward* his values for managing his diabetes, rather than *away* from his difficult feelings and thoughts.

What Are Your Pieces?

Let's take a minute and think about what your "pieces," particularly those related to your diabetes, might be. To do this, take out your diabetes journal or a piece of paper and write down all of the negative thoughts, feelings, memories, bodily sensations, and emotions you have about your diabetes. These should be all of the things that you don't really like to think about related to your diabetes, such as your fears, any shame or embarrassment that you have about having diabetes, thoughts or worries about your ability to take care of your diabetes, and any body changes or experiences you have noticed such as tingling feet, blurry vision, fatigue, or other symptoms that you do not like.

Now, on a separate column or page, write down all the positive thoughts, feelings, memories, bodily sensations, and emotions that you have to "combat" these negative emotions. For example, if you counter your fears about complications with the thought "But I feel good most of the time," write that down here. If you find yourself trying to bring up positive thoughts or feelings in order to keep your stress level down, write those thoughts and feelings in this section.

Now that you have a list of your red pieces and white pieces, imagine having all of these thoughts and feelings set on top of you as you lay flat on the ground as though you were a chessboard. See if you can see a distinction between you and each of these thoughts and feelings, whether they are positive or negative, without having to get rid of them or make them go away. Can you do it? This is a big step in moving toward your diabetes health rather than spinning your wheels trying to run away from your diabetes fears.

A Safe Place to Stand

One question our patients often ask at this point is why we would go through all this trouble to make a distinction between our "selves" and our "pieces." They wonder whether their pieces are just part of them, and if we're not going to try to get rid of them, why do we need to worry about whether they are something separate from their self or not. The answer is simple. The reason we talk about our thoughts, feelings, memories, and emotions as something separate from us is that it is from that place that we may be able to move on to the next step: actually being willing to let them be there. If our thoughts and feelings were undeniably true and were what defined us, we would certainly have to get rid of any that were negative or that we didn't like, right? But since your thoughts and feelings are "pieces" that you hold, not what makes up your true self, the task of noticing them is a lot less difficult.

Think back to Louis's story. There would probably be no way that Louis would be willing to let his urges be there and not have to eliminate their uncomfortable presence by eating some sweets after dinner, if his belief that he *had* to have something sweet was somehow really true and integral to who Louis was. Ironically, Louis really believed that he had to eliminate that urge in order to not eat sweets, but it was his noticing it as an urge and not something that was necessarily true or something that required getting rid of that finally allowed him to change his behavior.

It is one thing to understand why this noticing self would be helpful. It is another to experience it and to connect it to your life. In the next chapter we will provide additional experiences and exercises that will help expand your contact with this sense of "being the board" and help you see how it can empower the management of your diabetes.

Summing It Up

The way we conceptualize ourselves can sometimes cause us to get stuck in patterns that differ from our values.

Understanding your self as the place where your thoughts and feelings occur, rather than being made up of those thoughts and feelings, is a way to be able to notice them without having to eliminate them.

CHAPTER 6

Willing to *What?*

In the last chapter, we talked about perceiving a difference between your noticing self and your thoughts, feelings, and fears about diabetes. As we mentioned, the distinction is important because it can help you to create a place where you would be able to have all of your thoughts, fears, worries, and feelings about your diabetes without having to try to eliminate them. From this as a starting place, we now move on to trying out the idea of being willing to have *all* of your difficult thoughts and feelings about diabetes and life in general, even the ones it seems like you should try to avoid or eliminate.

At this point, it may not be very clear what we mean by "willing" or "willingness," so we'll spend some time here trying to describe how we're using these terms. Even if you understand what we mean by the words, however, it may not be that simple to do; many times being willing involves moving toward the very thing we're trying to move away from.

Defining Willingness

Let us start with a definition of the word "willing." Our understanding and use of the term in this context is originally from the work of Hayes, Strosahl, and Wilson (1999).

In your daily life, if you are willing to do something, it means that you will do it whether or not you want to. For instance, if you tell your spouse that you are willing to pick the kids up from school today, it usually means that even though you may not want to be the one to have to do it, you will do it because there is a larger purpose (larger than your desire or lack of desire) to doing it.

Willing and Wanting

We should notice here that willing does not mean the same as wanting, and that they are actually often opposites; you may be willing to do things that you are not wanting to do, like pick up the kids, or clean up a mess in the kitchen, or let your boss take credit for your hard work if it means keeping your job. Willing is not necessarily the same as "not wanting," though. If you absolutely do not want to do something, many times you are not willing to do it. For example, most of us would not be willing to commit a serious crime or bring harm to somebody we love, even if there seemed to be a good reason to do so.

The reasons why willing is not the same as wanting or not wanting are important to understanding what we mean by willingness. Because being willing is different from wanting, you don't necessarily have to want to do something to be willing to do it. Because being willing is different than not wanting, there is usually a higher purpose for why you would do it—higher than just your wants. You pick up the kids because you value their being brought home safely and you value not having too much pressure being put on your spouse. You clean up a mess because you value having a clean kitchen to safely prepare food in. You let your boss take credit for your work because you value having a job and maybe being a person who doesn't get too caught up in the credit.

Values, Values, Values

Noticing a theme here? When we break down areas where you might be willing (without necessarily wanting) to do or experience something, it is typically because there is a higher *value* held for doing or experiencing that thing. This is the same principle that we use when we talk about our values (see chapter 3) and taking care of diabetes. You may not *want* to do all of the things that are required to care for your diabetes—in fact, most people don't. And even with that being true, you can still do them, because you value being around to see your grandchildren graduate from high school, or you value being a person who takes good care of themselves.

Diabetes Computer

One way to think about how you might be willing to take care of your diabetes even if you do not want to is to think about what it would be like to have a computer that was all about your struggles (Hayes, Strosahl, and Wilson 1999). Maybe we can call this computer your "diabetes computer." This diabetes computer would work just like any other computer; it would have hardware and software and would take in input and give out output depending on the computation of that input with the software and hardware.

Input

When thinking about your diabetes computer, let's start with focusing on how this computer would get information in order to come up with output. Imagine if everybody you know were able to turn on your diabetes computer and type in whatever they wanted. Maybe some friends and family would type in supportive words and phrases of encouragement for the management of your diabetes. Maybe some would type in less supportive statements as well, like that you weren't doing a good job of managing your diabetes, or that they noticed you eating something you weren't supposed to or not taking care of your diabetes the way you should.

Now imagine that you also could add input into this computer. You would add some thoughts and feelings about your diabetes that were positive; maybe you would tell yourself that you could beat this disease or that you would do a great job of managing your diabetes from now on. And maybe some days you would add negative input into your diabetes computer. You might occasionally get discouraged and type in that you were never going to be able to manage your diabetes, or maybe you'd write about your worries about losing your feet or your eyesight or having other serious medical problems because of your diabetes.

Output

So whatever the input is, no matter how positive or negative, the computer would just take it all in, as computers do, and compute based on this input and its particular hardware and software. Now imagine that the computer does its computing and the output that pops up on the screen is: "Your diabetes is never going to be in control, and it will only get worse." How would you feel? Would you feel like giving up? Maybe you would find yourself hitting the "delete" button, trying to make this message go away. Or maybe you would find friends or family to blame, becoming angry with them or yourself. Maybe you would not want to look at the computer screen, or you would try the printer to see if the output there was different. But no matter what you did, the message would not go away or change, and everything you tried gave you the message "Your diabetes is never going to be in control, and it will only get worse."

This situation would probably feel pretty helpless. And maybe this is about what you were feeling when you picked up this book— like everything you tried just reminded you that you were stuck and overwhelmed by everything that needs to be done to manage this difficult disease.

Perspective

But what if there was one small thing that wouldn't take away the message on the screen but *would* change what it meant to you? The small thing would be your perspective of the computer screen. For example, imagine a person watching a suspenseful movie on their computer. They are holding their face very close to the computer screen and are very engrossed in what is showing. If something unexpected popped out from somewhere, they would probably jump as though the thing had popped out into the room with them. From this reaction, it could seem as though there were no computer screen there at all, and that the person was interacting with the things going on as though they were really there.

Now imagine somebody else is watching the same movie on their computer, but this time the person is sitting back a bit, and although they can see the movie and everything happening on their screen, they also can see the wall behind their computer, and maybe the papers stacked up on their desk. When something pops out on the screen, this person may notice it and react, but they may not jump quite as high, since they can see a little more clearly that what is happening on the screen is not happening in the same room with them.

How do you think these two people would react to a message coming in to the middle of their movie saying, "Your diabetes is never going to be in control, and it will only get worse"? Maybe the first person would feel as though they needed to do something to make that message go away. They may feel as though the message was meant for them, and that it was not something they wanted to see. The second person, on the other hand, might be surprised to see the message on the screen, but they may not have quite as strong a need to get rid of it. They may even have the thought, "Wow, how interesting. There's a sentence on the screen that could apply to me." But, because of their posture and how far they are sitting from the screen, they don't automatically assume that the message is true or is there in the room with them.

Our hope in this book is to help you make this shift in your perspective in terms of your own diabetes computer's messages. We'd like you to become more willing to have all kinds of messages and thoughts on the screen without having to change that output, in part because you are sitting back just a bit. We think that if we can do this, there will be less need for you to change what you're thinking and feeling, since you'll be sitting back far enough to see that just because they pop up on your screen doesn't necessarily mean that they are true.

I'm Having the Thought That ...

Many times at this point, people have one of two reactions. They either think, "Okay, I'm willing, let's go!" or they think, "Okay, I'm mostly willing … Well, I'm willing to have some experiences but not those really hard ones." Both reactions are, of course, completely normal. For most of us, the idea of being willing to have the really negative, deep-down scary stuff, like the thought that having diabetes could mean failing or even losing our life, is not acceptable because we're convinced that if we don't think about that or if we aren't really aware of what's down there, it seems not quite so scary.

One way to help balance this fear is to recall the idea of the noticing self we talked about in chapter 5. If we think of ourselves as the chessboard in the metaphor described there, rather than the pieces or the players, we have a safe place to stand where we could be willing to experience scary thoughts and feelings about having diabetes or other issues in our lives without having to get rid of them. From this space, we can notice our thoughts and feelings as just that: thoughts and feelings.

Another way to get into the space to do this is to label thoughts and feelings *as* thoughts and feelings (Hayes, Strosahl, and Wilson 1999). For example, if you had a loved one who had diabetes, and you watched them lose their vision and maybe experience an amputation, and you believed that the same would happen to you after you are diagnosed with diabetes, it would be a pretty scary situation. You may not be willing to have any thoughts about your diabetes because they would remind you of something that would be too hard to think about. What this resistance does, however, is automatically make your thoughts or worries true or believable, just because you're having them. In essence, all you have at this point is a fear or a belief that something bad will happen to you because you have been diagnosed with diabetes. But these are just thoughts, beliefs, and fears—not the truth. Look what happens when we label them as what they are:

"My father lost his vision and one of his feet because of his diabetes. I just found out that I have diabetes, and the same thing is going to happen to me."

vs.

"My father lost his vision and one of his feet because of his diabetes. I just found out that I have diabetes, and I have the worry that the same thing is going to happen to me."

Labeling thoughts as thoughts, feelings as feelings, beliefs as beliefs, worries as worries, and so on allows us to step back a little from what we're thinking and feeling—much like backing up from our computer screen. This act alone can sometimes be the most powerful move in freeing us up a little from what we're struggling with. For example, take the case of Scott, a sixty-seven-year-old retired schoolteacher who has been struggling with managing his diabetes for nearly twenty years. He told us that he doesn't have a hard time understanding what he needs to do to take care of his diabetes, but he has a very hard time getting himself to do it. He finds that every time he starts a new focus on his diet or exercise, the momentum only lasts a few days, and then he is right back where he started. Only, at that point, he also has feelings that he has failed again, and thoughts telling him that trying only makes things worse because he always ends up failing and then he feels bad about himself.

By the time Scott came to see us in the diabetes clinic, he had long since given up trying new things because of this cycle. In just a few minutes of talking, it became clear that Scott's biggest problem was not that he was having these thoughts that seemed to dictate that he shouldn't even try to take care of his diabetes, but that he *believed* them 100 percent. In fact, it made a lot of sense that he was having the thoughts; he had tried many times before and failed. But deciding that the thoughts were true was limiting his options for what he *could* do to turn things around. He was amazed that we weren't asking him not to feel these things and think these thoughts but just to notice that he was feeling and thinking them, and that they were feelings and thoughts and not necessarily the truth.

Remember, the purpose of not trying to eliminate these hard thoughts and feelings is not just for the fun of it, but so that you can be moving *toward* your diabetes values rather than *away* from these thoughts and feelings. Now that we have started the process of backing up a little from our thoughts and feelings, noticing them as just thoughts and feelings, we can put these skills together into a single practice.

Meditation Exercise

Virtually all spiritual and religious traditions practice one form or another of meditation. Because of this, meditation has become linked to the concept of religion. That is fine, but it has made the whole topic complicated and difficult when we are using it to promote health. That's unfortunate, because regular meditation practice has enormous health benefits. It is one of the very best ways to train your mental muscles to be present in the moment as the noticing you, letting go of avoidance and getting stuck in your thoughts. In effect, meditation is an extended willingness exercise that uses many of the skills we have worked with so far. The skills you practice in meditation can then be there to help you when difficult thoughts or feelings pop up unexpectedly.

We can simplify the healthy mental exercise of meditation into five simple steps. First we will list them and then expand on them and explain why they are needed.

1. Sit up straight and tall, preferably in an armless chair with a comfortable seat that you can sit in without touching the back.

2. Open your eyes and gaze down at about a 45 degree angle. Try to look at a neutral space about four feet away from you, something like the base of a blank wall.

3. Put one hand, palm up, in your lap. Put your other hand, palm up, in the palm of your first hand. Hold your upper arms and elbows so they are a little away from the trunk of your body and sit still.

4. Allow your awareness to settle on your breath. When your awareness wanders, gently allow it to come back to that focus.

5. Do this silently for at least five minutes, twice a day.

That's it. We mean it. That's it!

We can shorten the five rules to a sentence: For a few minutes twice a day, sit up tall and attentively with nothing to look at and nothing to feel other than noticing you are here, in your body, in this place.

Why would this be helpful? In essence we are giving your mind nothing to "work on" so that we can strengthen your ability to be an attentive, aware, noticing you. That way, you can use your analytical skills when they are helpful and learn to leave them be when they are not.

Problem solving leads naturally to your mind trying to change things. It spends its time figuring out how to get rid of what you do not like and how to produce what you do like. That is great when it works (as it does much of the time), but when you're experiencing difficult feelings or thoughts, these skills can run away with you. You forget who you are and you lose focus on what you are doing. You can find yourself back on autopilot.

Think back to the Overpass Exercise in the last chapter. The noticing you is standing under the overpass. The "thought" cars are speeding by above. Problem solving requires that you jump up into one of these cars. But once you do so you have gone from looking *at* the cars to looking out at the world *from* the cars. Once there, lots of things can no longer be seen clearly. Other cars whiz by so fast you can hardly see what they look like; trees are hard to distinguish; you can't risk gazing up at a cloud. And worse in some ways, lots of things now seem dangerous. For example, a car headed right toward you would look life threatening. You have lost your safe place.

The problem is that the human mind is such a powerful problem-solving organ that it virtually *demands* that you jump into one of the cars. So we need to create special situations that allow us to practice declining the invitation to do so.

Meditation is such a situation. Go back now to the five rules, and you can see why each and every one is there.

Sitting Up Straight and Tall

Most often meditation books will ask that you sit cross-legged on the floor. This position may be a bit better if you are flexible enough to do it, but there is a real risk of injury to your knees if you are not. Sitting in a chair will do fine, but it has to be done in a certain way. By "straight and tall" we mean with your spine straight and the very top of your head floating up toward the sky as if to touch it. This is a super way to improve your posture, though that is just a side effect. You are aligning yourself with gravity, and except for your feet and rear end, you are holding your body, rather than the chair or floor holding it. This is important because it takes attention and a little effort. If you slouch back into the chair you can quickly relax and lose focus. You can even fall sleep. Just relaxing, and even more so sleeping, is not meditation. You have to be awake, alert, and focused to learn how to decline your mind's invitations to avoidance and problem solving. Sitting straight and tall, without touching the back or arms of a chair, provides the structure to be awake and alert. It also gives you natural feedback. As soon as you start to lose your attention to the moment it is natural to start to slouch—which gives you rapid feedback that your attention has wandered away. You will notice that same purpose in some of the other rules.

Looking Down at the Wall

Keeping your eyes open is helpful for two reasons: it means you are aware of what is present in the world outside of your body (thus giving the noticing you something to be present with), and it (like sitting up straight and tall) helps keep you from going to sleep. But why not sit outside and look at the scenery or at least allow yourself to contemplate something beautiful? Wouldn't that be more relaxing? Actually there are meditation practices that are a little like that, but this one is simpler and safer. Unless it is done just right, giving your mind things to look at and evaluate goes against our purpose here. We ask that you look down at a 45 degree angle at the base of the wall for postural reasons—letting your head fall down can lead to sleeping and letting your head fall back produces unnecessary muscle tension. As for choosing a setting, any place that is quiet and where you will not be disturbed for five minutes or so will do. It is best to practice in the same place each time, at least at first, so you are not tempted to look around and generate lots of new opinions about your surroundings.

Hand in Hand, Arms Away

When you put one hand in another, palms up, your thumbs will naturally come together, putting you in a classic meditation posture. A common metaphor is to imagine you are holding a precious egg in your hands. This posture keeps your hands still and supported. If instead you let your arms move around, your mind would soon give your hands a task to accomplish (something like determining what the fabric on the chair feels like). And just like sitting straight and tall, keeping your hands like that and your arms just a fraction away from your body is an easy posture that still requires just enough attention to stay alert and focused. Experienced meditators often have their hands just a fraction above their laps, for much the same reason. You can decide for yourself what works best for you.

Breath In and Out, Twice a Day

Okay, we admit it. We combined the last two rules so that we could turn this whole section into a simple poem:

Sitting up, straight and tall.
Looking down, at the wall.
Hand in hand; arms away,
Breath in and out, twice a day.

The "focus on the breath" advice requires some additional explanation—otherwise we risk giving our minds another kind of problem to solve ("I need to focus on my breath! I'm not doing it! Oh no, whatever should I do?!"). Focusing on the breath is done gently and naturally, not forcefully and energetically. Much of the advice in this whole section comes from a wonderful little book on meditation by Raymond Reed Hardy (2000). He describes attending to your breath using the metaphor of a balloon settling into a funnel. When your attention wanders it is like the balloon being disturbed by a breeze and floating up. When you become aware and just get out of the way it will settle back down into the funnel like a golf ball on a tee. But if you energetically and forcefully try to control your attention it is like trying to get the balloon back into the funnel by flapping a fan at it to get it to float down. The balloon may go down, but it will only tend to bounce right out. Focusing on the breath allows you to attend, but it is self-defeating to create yet another problem to be solved.

It takes a while to begin to notice what meditation does to a human mind. Weeks, at least. But then, gradually, you will see change, which will deepen over time. Stress will be reduced; the ability to be present will increase; the sense of the noticing self will be much more real, and you will start to see how all of this interconnects with your ability to be willing—to say yes to what life gives you—and to keep moving in a valued direction. The effect is like looking out of your window at your yard with the clutter removed. Somehow the underbrush is no longer there. Things just seem clearer.

It is best not to turn your expectations or the changes you in fact see into yet another problem. If not much happens, great. If a lot happens, great. In either case, just thank your mind for its opinions and come back to the simple purpose of sitting. The advice to do this for just a few minutes twice a day is designed to keep you doing it and to keep you humble. Start with five minutes and don't increase it much for a few weeks, at least. Meditation is not a new problem-solving technique. It is an exercise, like stretching or jogging. Quickly trying to meditate for long periods is a sure sign that you are forcing the issue.

Just like with any new activity, you may find that meditating brings up some new anxiety in the beginning. Again, this is okay. In fact, really noticing and being willing to feel your anxiety when it is there is one of the keys to being able to live fully in your values. In fact, the following section will help you to think about why *looking for* anxiety might be a good thing.

Finding Anxiety

When we experience anxiety, most of us do just about everything we can think of to end it or make it stop. We might try to distract ourselves with a book or by watching television, or we might try to solve whatever problem is causing the anxiety or find some way to make it go away. So far in this book we have talked about why this might not work and why it might cause more problems to try to deny or not think about these things.

A slightly different way to think about this, though, is to think about the advantage of actually doing things to try to *find anxiety*. Many times when we bring up this idea to patients they get a look in their eye that tells us that they think we have finally lost it. But the purpose of thinking about anxiety this way is to keep the focus on moving in the direction of your values, rather than away from negative thoughts and feelings.

The exercise below is a chance to do just that—to come up with an activity that will bring all of these thoughts and feelings up for you, so that you can practice responding differently to them and moving in the direction of your values.

Willingness Exercise

When we talked about willingness earlier, we made a distinction between being willing to do something and wanting to do it. Typically, that distinction makes a lot of sense to our patients; they usually understand from the experiences in their own life that they don't always want to do the things that need doing, but they are willing to do them anyway to meet a larger goal. That distinction is the most clear, however, when we talk about actually implementing the idea of willingness into their lives by going in search of anxiety to practice being willing to experience it.

In this exercise, adapted loosely from Hayes, Strosahl, and Wilson (1999), our objective is to find something small for you to do that will help clarify the distinction between willingness and wanting while starting the process of moving you toward your values. To do this, you should spend some time thinking about some small goal or action you can set for yourself that is related to your values but is just outside of your comfort zone. For example, if you value being a person who contributes to your community but have never had the time, organization, or the self-confidence to call up a local organization and find an event or cause to take part in, this is the opportunity to take that step.

Maybe you are living your values in many areas of your life but are primarily struggling in the area of your diabetes. If so, think about your diabetes management and see if there is an area that you are not as consistent as you would like to be. For example, do you consistently take your medication or insulin, or do you sometimes forget and need to make adjustments to try to compensate? Or do you pay pretty good attention to your medication and diet but struggle with fitting exercise into your daily life? Or do you know that your eating has caused problems and contributed to excess weight and increased blood glucose over the years, but you are unsure where to start to change some of your habits?

All of these areas, plus all of the areas we talked about in chapter 3 when we discussed your values, are fair game. The objective within whichever area you choose, then, is to come up with a small but important step you can take in the direction of that value. The step should involve some degree of stretch for you; remember that our objective here also is to give you the opportunity to experience thoughts and feelings that you might ordinarily try to avoid, like anxiety or urges to eat, drink, or engage in behaviors that are not consistent with your diabetes management. The emphasis here is on finding a step that is both small enough that you can actually implement it, but large enough that it will bring up some of the thoughts and feelings that we want to practice willingness with. If your diet is out of control, the place to start would not be to overhaul every food that you eat or reduce your calorie intake to 500 per day, because you would probably not be able to sustain such a change. Likewise, it wouldn't be a very significant change to say that instead of six cookies after dinner each night, you will reduce it to five, because while this is a change in the right direction, it's not likely to bring up uncomfortable thoughts, feelings, or urges for you to practice noticing.

One patient, Jessica, had a difficult time coming up with a goal for her willingness exercise. She was a thirty-eight-year-old, single, overweight woman who had been diagnosed with diabetes a year earlier and had not yet gotten her blood glucose under control. When we started talking with her, we found that this was just one of the things she was struggling with. Her weight had made her feel very self-conscious, and she had never had a serious relationship because she was afraid to put herself into social situations where she might meet somebody. She had a number of friends and a good job, but her weight and her lack of a partner were constant stressors for her, and she found that staying in her apartment and eating were the main ways she coped with her situation.

When we asked her to come up with this first act of willingness, she first said that she would try to lose fifteen pounds as a starting place for the one hundred and twenty pounds she hoped to lose. While we liked the idea of her finding a smaller target than her overall weight-loss goal, the target of losing fifteen pounds didn't tell us much about what she wanted to *change* in her life. For example, we didn't know if she would lose the fifteen pounds by starving herself or by eating only chocolate chip cookies (if needed, see chapter 7 for a description of why this is not a good idea!). We also didn't know how her weight loss related to her values. When we spent some time breaking it down with her, we found that her actual value was to be a healthy person who cared about what she put into her body. She felt that more than weight loss, highlighting and living that value would allow her to pursue relationships and move forward in her life.

With the value in mind, she changed her willingness goal to eating at least three servings of vegetables every day. This was less than she hoped to be eating long-term, but it was consistent with her value of being a person who put healthy things into her body. It was an achievable first step, and it would give her the opportunity to notice uncomfortable thoughts and feelings when she had to make a choice between potato chips and a green salad at her favorite lunch restaurant.

Just like with Jessica, your objective is to find a goal that is both accomplishable and important to your values. In addition, it should be a goal that requires you to feel or experience a thought, sensation, or urge that ordinarily would serve as a barrier to your attempting the action. Think about it for a minute, and then write down in your diabetes journal what you will be attempting. Remember that some actions, like taking the first step in a relationship that has become distant, will be one-time actions, whereas others, like incorporating exercise into your life, will be more permanent. That doesn't mean that there won't be days that you can't reach the goal you set, but the idea is to continue moving in the direction of your values.

Now write down what thoughts, feelings, or urges you'll need to be willing to have in order to do this.

Based on our experience, there are a few suggestions that may make initiating and maintaining this new behavior easier and more consistent. Make sure to give yourself a timeline for accomplishing tasks that occur once, and a timeline for making a habit of tasks that occur every day or every week. For example, if your goal is to reconnect with a friend or family member you have become disconnected from, be sure to set a date by which you want to make the initial contact. And if your goal is to incorporate a daily activity, like exercise, into your life, you may want to start with a few days a week and work up to exercising daily. Additionally, make sure that you tell close friends and family members of your plans and ask for their support in carrying out the new behaviors until they become a habit (see chapter 13 for a discussion of why talking about it matters). Finally, don't give up! For almost any new behavior there is a period of time when it feels too hard to pull off or when the old behavior shows up again. That's okay. Just make sure that you notice all the thoughts and feelings that go along with this new wrinkle, and get back on the path to willingness.

Summing It Up

Being willing to have negative thoughts and feelings is not the same as wanting to have them.

To be willing, you need to learn to look at *your mind, not just* from *your mind.*

Willingness involves taking steps that feel scary or difficult so that you can live your values more fully.

PART III

Your Individual Diabetes Plan

CHAPTER 7

Food, Glorious Food

Ah, food. Food is undoubtedly the most complicated aspect of managing your diabetes. Entire books are written about the diabetes diet: what you should do, what you shouldn't do, how to count calories, carbohydrates, and fat grams, as well as strategies for getting the most out of the foods that you do eat and minimizing the foods that can raise your blood glucose too high. Theories and fads are introduced and tested; diets high in carbohydrates or low in carbohydrates, high in fat or low in fat, high in protein or low in protein. Given the vast amount of information out there, we won't try to educate you about all of the things you could possibly learn about eating and diabetes, and we won't try to tell you what will be the best diet for you. Instead, the purpose of this chapter is to highlight what is known about eating and diabetes and to teach you how to find out what works best for your body so that you can *live your values for managing your diabetes*. In other words, if you have the value of being a healthy, fit person who takes care of their diabetes, either as its own value or so that you can see your children get married or your grandchildren graduate from high school, we want to help you establish an individualized plan for how to do that, which includes a focus on the most important aspects of managing your diet.

Diabetes Diet Basics

One of the most difficult aspects of managing a diabetes diet is the plain fact that no matter what your relationship with food has been up until now, and even if eating has led to weight and health problems, you still have to eat. If you had a different type of problem, like drinking too much or smoking, the recommendation most doctors and health care professionals would make would be that you give up drinking or smoking altogether rather than trying to cut down or to continue but to change your amount of drinking or smoking.

But you can't give up eating. Even if eating the wrong foods has contributed to developing diabetes or other health problems, or if your eating habits have led to gaining more weight than is recommended, food is not something you can quit altogether. Instead, taking care of your diabetes requires that you learn and keep a new set of eating habits. To start on the road to these new habits, we first have to understand the purpose of the different types of foods we eat every day.

The Role of Carbohydrates

Carbohydrates are an energy source that comes in many types of foods, and that is responsible for most of the rise in glucose in the bloodstream that leads to problems in diabetes. There are three main types of carbohydrates: 1) starches (or complex carbohydrates), 2) sugars, and 3) fiber. These three sources vary in their roles in the body, but they all follow generally the same process when it comes to blood sugar. Whatever the source of the carbohydrates, the body breaks them down into simple sugars, which are absorbed into the bloodstream in the intestines. Once this sugar is in the bloodstream, insulin is normally produced in the pancreas automatically. The insulin enters the bloodstream and acts as a "key" for opening up cells and muscle tissue to let the broken-down carbohydrate energy into the cells to provide power for the cell to function. If insulin is not produced or is not working properly in the system, the blood sugar energy remains in the bloodstream, which leads to complications (see chapter 11). Below is a description of each of the types of carbohydrates in detail.

Starches

Carbohydrates considered to be "starches" are found in many foods. Vegetables such as potatoes, peas, and corn; legumes such as dried beans, lentils, kidney and pinto beans, and black-eyed and split peas; and grains such as rice, oats, and barley all are considered starches. These foods can be either *whole grain*, where the entire kernel of the grain is contained in the food, or *refined grain*, where many of the nutrients and fiber are removed, leaving only the starchy portion of the grain. Needless to say, whole-grain foods tend to be the more nutritious of the two. It is sometimes difficult to tell the difference, however, between foods that are whole grain and those which are refined, so it is important to look at the label of the food if you are unsure whether it's whole grain or not. Whole-grain foods will have as the first ingredient either whole-wheat flour, brown rice, rye flour, barley, or oats.

Many people, including the American Diabetes Association, advocate for diets high in starches for individuals with diabetes. The reason for this is that these foods contain very little fat, saturated fat, or cholesterol, and the whole-grain varieties often contain vitamins, minerals, and fiber (see discussion on fiber below). Carbohydrates in general, however, have been the source of much debate in the diabetes diet world: they raise your blood glucose more quickly than proteins and fats, but they contain many of the components needed to maintain a healthy diet, heart, and weight.

Sugars

Sugar has long been considered the natural-born enemy of the person with diabetes. This is largely because diabetes was thought of as a disease of too much sugar in the body, and for years people thought that eating too much sugar would cause a person to develop diabetes. We now know that diabetes is not caused by excess sugar, but the issue of whether foods high in sugar can contribute to blood sugar problems is not quite as clear-cut. On the one hand, our bodies turn all carbohydrates into sugars in the body, so it is the total amount of carbohydrates of any kind consumed that makes the biggest difference in blood sugar levels. On the other hand, we now know that some foods, and particularly those foods high in sugar and refined grains, have a more profound impact on blood sugar levels than others (see discussion of glycemic index below).

Whatever the impact of sugar on the body, in recent years dieticians and doctors have realized that telling an individual with diabetes to eliminate sugar from their diet is not generally very realistic: people tend to eat sugar whether they are told not to or not. Now sugar is often recommended as a special treat for people with diabetes—something to use sparingly and on special occasions, that is added to an overall healthy diet and eaten in the place of a similar carbohydrate such as potatoes or rice. Calories present in sugar, of course, always need to be considered, in cases where weight loss is a health goal.

Sugar is present in foods either naturally or as an added ingredient to sweeten. It is found naturally in milk and fruits, and is added to foods ranging from ketchup to cookies in order to enhance flavor. When sugar is found in milk it is called *lactose* and in fruits it is called *fructose*. In fact, just about any ingredient in a food that ends in "ose" is technically a sugar.

Sugar Substitutes

Sugar substitutes are seen as a way for people to maintain their sweet tooth without overdoing it on their sugar consumption. While many sugar substitutes exist on the market today that do the job of sweetening food without sugar, it is important to remember that many foods sweetened with sugar substitutes often still contain high levels of refined carbohydrates, and thus similar restraint needs to be used in consuming them as would be required with sugar. For instance, sugar-free candy should not be confused with a food that is healthful or one that should be consumed with abandon, given that these candies often still contain high levels of carbohydrates just like regular candy. Sweeteners used in coffee, such as saccharin and aspartame, often do not contain high levels of carbohydrates, but certain types are not recommended for pregnant or nursing mothers (saccharin) or individuals with phenylketonuria (aspartame).

Fiber

Fiber is an important part of our diets that comes from plant foods such as whole grains, legumes, nuts, and certain fruits and vegetables. Although considered a carbohydrate in the United States, fiber is considered a separate category of food in many countries in the world. It is broken down into soluble and insoluble fiber, each of which serves important functions in the body.

Soluble fiber is found in fruits, legumes, vegetables, and seeds. It is very important in a diabetes diet because it slows down and reduces absorption of glucose in the intestines.

Insoluble fiber is found in bran, whole grains, and nuts. This type of fiber is important to good colon functioning, in that it helps to clean out the gastrointestinal tract and keep waste moving through the body.

In addition to these advantages, fiber can also make you feel fuller after eating, an advantage to individuals trying to lose weight or watch portion sizes or snacking. The benefits of fiber are clear. However, it is often difficult for people, whether they have diabetes or not, to get enough fiber in their diets. The recommended amount of fiber per day is 25 to 35 grams; most Americans get just under half that amount.

The Role of Proteins

Proteins are an energy source made up of amino acids and used in the body for fuel. Much of the protein we get in our diets is made up of meat, eggs, or milk from animals, as well as an increasing amount from soy and other plants. When our protein comes from animal sources, the fat content of the food needs to be considered, since these foods tend to be higher in fat (see discussion of fats below). Most experts recommend that people with diabetes eat between 10 and 30 percent of their calories from protein. This number varies widely depending on the food plan, the source of protein (plant or animal), and the fat content, but for many years the recommendation was for people with diabetes to limit their protein intake to a reasonably small level.

The reasons for this limitation were twofold. First, because protein sources from animals tend to be higher in fat than carbohydrates, reducing protein is considered important in preventing heart disease and other problems that are worsened by high levels of saturated fat and cholesterol. While this consideration has likely led to a decrease in complications of this sort, newer preparations of protein generated from soy products have made this somewhat less problematic.

Another consideration for individuals with diabetes when determining their level of protein intake is the potentially damaging effect of protein on the kidneys. Several studies have demonstrated this effect on impaired kidneys, but there is still debate about whether protein has a damaging effect on nonimpaired kidneys, and whether a diet that is low in protein protects kidney function any better than a high-protein food plan.

The Role of Fats

Like carbohydrates, there are multiple types of fats that need to be considered when talking about fat's role in a diabetes diet. Most experts agree that fats should not make up more than about 30 percent of a person's diet, whether they have diabetes or not, and that the types of fat that contribute most to the development of heart disease should be used as little as possible.

Cholesterol

Cholesterol is a type of fat that most people are at least generally familiar with. Excess cholesterol in the body contributes both to coronary artery disease and the development of strokes (see chapter 11), and therefore it is recommended that cholesterol intake should be limited in people at risk for developing these problems, such as individuals with diabetes. The general recommendation is no more than 300 milligrams a day.

Saturated Fat

Saturated fat is a type of fat that generally comes from animal products; meats, cheese, and eggs are some of the primary culprits. This type of fat is considered "bad fat" in that it contributes to the development of heart disease more than unsaturated fat. Saturated fat increases the cholesterol levels in your blood, which can contribute to heart attacks and strokes.

Unsaturated Fat

Unlike saturated fats, which come from animal sources, unsaturated fats come from vegetables. Unsaturated fats such as olive oil and margarine historically have been considered better for you than saturated fats. In actuality, we are really talking about two different types of fats when we talk about unsaturated fats, since they are also broken down into two separate groups: monounsaturated and polyunsaturated.

Monounsaturated fats are the healthiest option in some opinions, because they do not raise cholesterol levels like saturated fats do, and thus appear to lead to less cardiovascular disease. This type of fat is found in canola oil, olive oil, many types of nuts, and avocados.

Polyunsaturated fats also do not raise cholesterol, but this type of fat, found in things like mayonnaise and margarine, does have a tendency to lower HDL or "good" cholesterol levels, which has a negative impact on heart health as well. Matters are complicated, however, by the fact that polyunsaturated fats appear to be protective against insulin resistance while monounsaturated fats appear to contribute to this problem that may lead to diabetes in some people (Lovejoy 2002).

Trans Fat

Finally, the newest and most talked-about type of fat these days is what is called *trans-fatty acid* or *trans fat* for short. These fats occur naturally in animal products in very small amounts, but the most common form of them available now is created by taking polyunsaturated fats and heating them up and adding hydrogen. The result, which was originally marketed as "shortening" in 1911, is an oil with the consistency of butter. This allows food manufacturers and fast-food restaurants to substitute this cheaper alternative in recipes that call for butter.

Trans fats are not thought to be beneficial to the body in any way, and appear to contribute to heart disease by raising LDL (bad) cholesterol while lowering HDL (good) cholesterol. They are found in commercially prepared foods such as donuts, baked goods, margarines, and many types of fast foods.

Test, Test, Test

The only sure way to know how your body reacts to carbohydrates, proteins, and fats is to monitor your blood sugar after eating different types of foods. To do this, you should check your blood glucose right before eating a meal and then one-and-a-half to two hours later and compare the two values. The difference between the two numbers will tell you how much your blood glucose increased due to the foods you ate.

Types of Diabetes Diets

Sometimes it seems as though for every person with diabetes, there is a new diet recommendation. These diets range from the old, no-nonsense food plans recommended by the Food and Drug Administration to newer, trendy approaches that base their recommendations on one or two ideas. Whatever the approach, it is clear that the maze of diet recommendations for diabetes is not always an easy thing to navigate, so we have given you a brief overview of the four main types of eating plans out there for people with diabetes.

Low-Fat, High-Carbohydrate Diets

For many years, diets low in fat and high in complex carbohydrates have been the standard recommendation for people with diabetes. These diets are embodied in the USDA's Food Pyramid and are extended in the Diabetes Pyramid recommended by the American Diabetes Association (see figure below). This type of food plan primarily emphasizes the role of fiber and unprocessed carbohydrates in the long-term maintenance of blood glucose levels and the prevention of heart-related complications.

Many people wonder, when first diagnosed with diabetes and looking at this food plan, how it can be that if they are experiencing a problem characterized by too much blood glucose, which is manufactured in the body from carbohydrates, the recommendation is to increase the amount of carbohydrates they take in. And in actuality, following a low-fat, high-carbohydrate diet has been shown to increase postmeal blood glucose. The reason for this recommendation lies more in what this type of food plan helps prevent. First, for people with insulin resistance, or an inability of the body to efficiently use existing insulin, a diet high in carbohydrates and low in fat is thought

Diabetes Pyramid

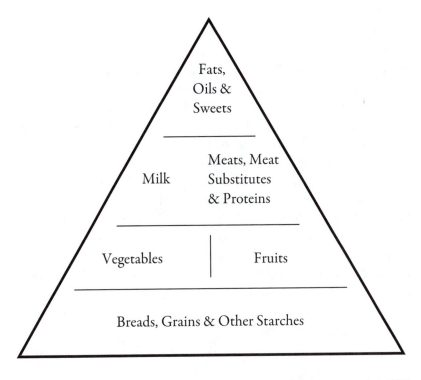

Fats,
Oils &
Sweets

Milk

Meats, Meat
Substitutes
& Proteins

Vegetables

Fruits

Breads, Grains & Other Starches

to reduce insulin resistance, thereby improving the body's long-term ability to utilize its own insulin.

Secondly, for either people with or without diabetes, diets low in fat have been shown to decrease the risk of heart disease. This is particularly important for individuals with diabetes, who might be at higher risk already due to their diabetes.

Low-Carbohydrate Diets

In recent years, there has been a lot of attention paid to diets low in carbohydrates. These diets, which typically advocate high protein and moderate fat intake levels, are essentially the reverse of the low-fat, high-carbohydrate diet described above. The majority of calories (about 40 to 70 percent, depending on the specific diet plan) come from protein sources. How the rest of the calories are divided up is dependent on the purposes of the diet: carbohydrate counts are very low for people who are also trying to lose weight and higher for those who are using the diet to keep posteating glucose levels low.

While these diets have been criticized widely for turning the USDA's Food Pyramid on its head, the basic premise behind these diets is consistent with the goals of managing blood glucose. By limiting the amount of carbohydrate taken in, studies have shown that an overall reduction in blood glucose levels can be achieved with these diets (for instance, Stern et al. 2004), particularly postmeal levels, which may be particularly important to good diabetes management (Temelkova-Kurktschiev et al. 2000).

By far, the biggest complaint lodged against low-carbohydrate, high-protein diets has been the effect of this type of plan on the development and exacerbation of heart disease. Because these diets tend to include higher levels of fat and cholesterol than low-fat, high-carbohydrate diets, people predisposed to or suffering from heart disease (and people with diabetes are often considered at high risk for cardiovascular conditions; see discussion in chapter 11) are typically thought to benefit more from a diet lower in fat and cholesterol. However, many assert that the weight loss and glucose benefits outweigh the potential risks associated with these plans.

Low-Glycemic-Index Diets

Another type of diet that has received increased attention lately is the low-glycemic-index diet. This diet is similar to the low-carbohydrate, high-protein diet, but instead of focusing on carbohydrates overall, this plan utilizes information about the effect of different types of food on blood glucose to emphasize the reduction of foods that have a higher likelihood of sending your blood glucose soaring.

For the past decade, scientists have been testing the actual effect of particular foods on a person's blood glucose by testing the body's reaction to different types of food. This process generally involves giving a group of people a specific food and then waiting a prescribed amount of time, then testing everybody's blood glucose levels and comparing the results to a test done on those same people with a standardized amount of glucose. Given that we know that all carbohydrates are not created equal in their impact on blood glucose levels, tests of this sort allow scientists to examine the actual effect on the blood glucose, rather than just the carbohydrate count, of real people. Once the tests have been completed on a large enough group of people, the results are averaged and this gives us a *glycemic value* for each food tested. Diets utilizing this information then recommend eating more foods with a low glycemic value and fewer foods with a high glycemic value.

While the relationship between glycemic value and blood glucose cannot be debated, there are still criticisms of this approach. One is that many foods that are commonly eaten have not yet been tested, so no glycemic value exists for them yet. Another is that this approach may give some people the feeling that they can eat large amounts of low-glycemic foods without consequences. While this type of false dieting security is generally a bad idea (we sometimes call it the "nonfat cookie syndrome"), it may be a particularly bad idea when it relies on the glycemic value of the food, because foods may vary significantly from one subtype to another. For example, there may be big glycemic differences between different types of potatoes, but a glycemic value is just computed for potatoes generally. Also, different people may have very different blood glucose reactions to the same food, since the glycemic value is just an average of what was found in the group of people tested.

Diabetes Exchange Diets

The fourth type of food plan popularly recommended to individuals with diabetes is the diabetes exchange or exchange list diet. This type of food plan allows a little bit of every type of food but requires an overall calorie limit and structure that requires fewer high-calorie foods or more low-calorie foods. For example, if a person should be eating a recommended 1,800 calories a day and is placed on an exchange diet, they are given a list of the portion sizes that constitute a serving for each food and a specified number of servings from each category (meat, dairy, starch, vegetables, etc.). Thus, they can eat whichever foods they want, but a serving for chocolate cake will be much smaller than a serving of spinach, and according to their calorie requirements they will only have a certain number of servings per day.

Exchange diets have long been criticized for being too complicated for real people to follow in their daily lives; but newer, more commercial versions of this same principle (such as the Weight Watchers Points program) have become very popular in recent years. Diabetes versions tend to contain about 60 percent carbohydrate, 10 to 20 percent protein, and less than 30 percent fat. However, given the wide flexibility in these plans, these numbers are often targets rather than what is actually consumed.

A Word About Portion Sizes

No matter which diabetes diet matrix you fall under, it is important to always think about the size of the meal you are eating and the impact of that meal on your diabetes. In the Western world, eating habits have changed dramatically over the years, and the size of our portions is only one example of how these eating habits can have disastrous effects on diabetes. However you divide up your carbohydrates, proteins, and fats throughout the day, paying attention to the portion size designated on the food label and splitting a meal or taking half home for leftovers when eating out are easy ways to keep portions in check. This will not only help your overall blood glucose levels but will also aid in taking off unneeded pounds, which very well may enhance your body's ability to manage your blood sugar as well.

Weight for It

Because of the way diabetes develops, it is not uncommon for people with type 2 diabetes to have struggles with their weight that were around long before their diabetes showed up. Sometimes this means that you have five or ten extra pounds, and sometimes it means that you have quite a bit more that you want or need to lose. In either case, being overweight is an incredibly difficult experience for many of us and not one that is tackled easily.

There are many aspects of losing weight that make it difficult to take (and keep) off unwanted pounds. Given the focus of this book and our backgrounds, we will focus more on the psychological elements that make it difficult. We will also come back to some practical ways to apply the things you have learned so far in this book to both managing your diabetes and targeting your weight if those are goals for you.

Motivation

One key complaint we hear all the time from patients who want to lose weight is that it's nearly impossible to keep up enough motivation to have the type of weight loss they would like to see. It might be helpful to think for a second about what motivation is and how we use it in our daily lives. We would define *motivation* as what people feel when they are accomplishing what they want to accomplish—when they are living their values (see chapter 3). Most people think that they need to feel motivated in order to meet their goals and make consistent changes in their behavior. If we think about it, though, there are often times when we don't feel motivated at all, and yet we still meet our goals and obligations. For example, there might be many days that you don't feel motivated to get up to go to work or school, or when you don't feel like making dinner or running errands. Yet, when these are things you feel you need to do, you are generally able to do them whether you feel motivated or not.

Another way to think about motivation is that it is just what you feel sometimes before and during the actual activity; that rather than causing you to be able to do something, it just happens to be there sometimes while you are doing it. If we think about motivation this way, it's easier to think about how you might be able to make changes to your eating habits even when you don't feel particularly motivated. In other words, motivation might just be one more chess piece that can be there or not, and your chessboard can still move forward regardless.

Shame

Another psychological aspect of being overweight and weight loss that doesn't get covered very often in all the diet books out there is shame. *Shame* is a feeling that many people experience in response to needing to lose weight. It combines feeling embarrassed about one's weight and feeling bad about oneself for being in a position where weight loss is suggested. Shame is an incredibly important part of the process of making changes in our weight because there is such a strong temptation to believe that it is true (that there actually is something wrong or bad about you) or to try to avoid it. Both of those processes make weight more difficult to deal with. When we believe our shame, we are basically believing the thought that we are somehow bad (and what would you expect in terms of success from a bad person?). When we try avoiding shame, we often become mindless about food and exercise.

Take Candice's example. Candice was a patient who came to our clinic stating that her doctor had told her that she needed to lose weight for her health. She had been to a nutritionist and had developed a good meal plan that she was happy with, but she found that no matter what she did, she kept gaining weight rather than losing it.

When we looked carefully at what and when Candice ate, we realized that she tended to stick to her meal plan, but she would eat much bigger portions when she was feeling vulnerable or embarrassed about herself. When we spent some time talking about why that was the case, Candice told us that she had a lot of shame about her appearance and would generally do whatever she could to make that shame go away as soon as she started to experience it. She said that one way to distract herself from it was to have a little more food, which always made her feel better, and she would eventually forget about her feelings of shame. As she was describing her situation to us, Candice said that she couldn't believe how much her story sounded like a person with an addiction to drugs or alcohol; she was using food to try to change her feelings rather than letting her feelings be there. With this awareness, we were able to help her notice her shame, from the position of her noticing self, rather than needing to eliminate it. This allowed her to stick to her diet (an action that was in line with her values) even when the shame was very strong.

It's important to note that not all people with extra weight to lose experience high levels of shame about their weight, and our discussion about shame is not to indicate that overweight people *should* feel ashamed, or that extra weight is something to be ashamed of. Rather, we bring it up here because a large percentage of our patients do report struggling with this emotion, and it is important to notice that shame is just like any other thought or feeling and does not need to be escaped from. The methods in this book apply perfectly to it.

Filling the Need

The last aspect of weight loss that needs to be addressed is the psychological need that food may potentially be meeting, and how that need will be addressed if changes are made in your diet. As noted above, for Candice, the need being met was to distract her from her feelings of shame and embarrassment. For other people the need might be to reduce stress at the end of a long day or after a difficult interaction, or to relieve boredom when there is nothing else to do. Some people report that eating rich or sweet foods helps reduce the urge or craving that might occur for these types of foods. It is important to remember that in each of these situations, the underlying purpose of the eating is to make a thought or feeling go away, rather than to notice it and move forward. Using your noticing-self skills or thinking about these thoughts and feelings as pieces on the chessboard will help in the long term to change the way you react to these thoughts and feelings. But in the short term, it's important that you have handy alternative ways of dealing with specific situations for when these occasions arise.

One way we talk about this with our patients is that noticing or being mindful of thoughts and feelings is like building a muscle—the more you use it, the stronger it will be. In the beginning, then, when the muscle is not that strong, it's a good idea to have a backup plan for what you are going to do if you have a stressful day, or for those days when you are bored with nothing to do. For example, if you have a difficult interaction with your spouse, and normally the first thing you would do is to head for the ice cream, you might want to figure out ahead of time a friend you can call to chat with or go take a walk with so that you don't have to face the temptation of the ice cream in the moment when you're experiencing stress.

Blood Sugar Levels and Diet

When we talk about diet, it is important to include a conversation about blood sugar levels, given that the foods we eat have the biggest influence on our blood sugar. If you have made it this far in this book, you probably already know the effects of low blood sugar, but a review might be helpful.

Hypoglycemia

Hypoglycemia refers to the condition of not having enough glucose in your blood and the problems that result from that state. Even people who don't have diabetes can have a version of hypoglycemia if they haven't eaten in too long or have been doing something that has used up all of their blood sugar, like vigorous exercise.

In diabetes, hypoglycemia is a short-term complication that results from something that is lowering your blood glucose. This is often the result of taking too much diabetes medication or insulin, but it can be caused by eating too little food or exercising too much. It should be noted that, particularly for people with type 2 diabetes, this is not necessarily a rare event, but it is a unique one, in that diabetes means that your body produces *too much* glucose and it has problems and complications as a result of that extra glucose. Therefore, to have a complication that is due to having too little glucose typically means that you have eaten too little for the amount of medication or insulin you have taken, since these medicines work to bring your blood glucose levels down to the levels of somebody without diabetes.

Symptoms of hypoglycemia sometimes feel like anxiety, such as sweating, rapid heartbeat, palpitations, skin becoming pale or white, and feeling anxious or panicky. Other times they feel like they are concentrated in your brain, with problems such as headache, fatigue, confusion, vision problems, and loss of concentration. When the symptoms are related more to your brain functioning, there is also a chance of having convulsions or entering into a coma. Thus, it's important to understand exactly what is happening with your blood glucose when you start to experience symptoms, and to treat it accordingly.

Treating Hypoglycemia

When hypoglycemia occurs, it is important to attend to it quickly in order to more serious complications from occurring. Eating or drinking something that will provide easily accessible glucose is the primary recommendation for hypoglycemia. Drugstores sell glucose tablets that you can carry with you for hypoglycemic moments. Two or three of these, or a couple of pieces of candy, or a small amount of sugary soda or orange juice will usually do the job of raising your glucose up to the correct levels.

One good idea is to test your blood sugar before you administer the sweets, if the symptoms aren't too severe. This will let you know what level your blood sugar is when you start to have symptoms. However, if you're feeling at all confused or if the symptoms feel strong, skip the testing and go right to administering the sweets. Then, regardless of your ability to test before the sweets, test your sugar about twenty minutes after the sweets to ensure that your levels have gone back to normal.

Hyperglycemia

Hyperglycemia is basically the opposite of hypoglycemia; it is what happens in your body when you have too much blood glucose. As you know, too much blood glucose is generally the problem with diabetes, so this is probably not a new experience for most people with diabetes, and these symptoms might have led to you finding out about your diabetes to begin with. However, it's still important to identify these symptoms so you can respond appropriately when they occur.

The symptoms of hyperglycemia include sleepiness, dry mouth, frequent urination, fatigue, and extreme thirst. Although these symptoms are not the same as those experienced in hypoglycemia, patients often confuse these symptoms with low blood sugar and may take glucose tablets or eat or drink something high in sugar to combat the supposed hypoglycemic event. Not surprisingly, this can cause pretty big problems when the problem really is blood sugar that is too high. Thus, if the symptoms aren't too severe, it's always a good idea to test your blood sugar before you administer something to increase it, in order to prevent confusing the two.

In this chapter we've discussed a range of diet topics to help you manage your diabetes and prevent complications through changes in what you eat. Clearly with a problem like diabetes, this is an important area to target, but it is not the only place to make changes. In the next chapter, we will discuss the important considerations for incorporating exercise into your life as well. This will help you fully understand the keys to great diabetes management so that as you think about setting goals and moving toward your values, the road map is clear.

Summing It Up

The foods we eat are broken down into carbohydrates, proteins, and fats, all of which can affect blood sugar levels and diabetes complications.

There are many types of diets recommended for diabetes, and the right one for you depends on your specific blood glucose goals and complication risks.

CHAPTER 8

Exercise Your Rights

We often ask patients the following questions when approaching the topic of exercise: "What if there was a pill that you could take that would help lower your risk for cardiovascular disease, help you lose weight, and help you keep that weight off? And what if that pill would also help you look more like you wanted to look? And what if it would lower your bad cholesterol and triglycerides and raise your good cholesterol? At the same time it would help lower your blood pressure, reduce your stress, reduce your need for insulin and diabetes medications, and in some cases bring your blood sugar levels down to those of a person without diabetes. Would you take it?"

Almost every person with diabetes we have ever asked this question of has said that they would take this pill immediately. So we ask, "What if you had to travel a long way to get the drug, and you could only go on foot, and you would have to go and get it multiple times a week? Would you still want it?" Again, people are generally still enthusiastic, since this mysterious drug seems to address so many problems experienced by people with diabetes. Then, when we tell them that rather than a drug, we are talking about exercise, almost universally, people are less excited.

There is something about the goal of consistent exercise that seems to feel insurmountable to people both with and without diabetes. In fact, when we do workshops or trainings for professionals on using this treatment approach, or when we meet with groups of people with or without diabetes for the first time, we always ask how many people get the recommended amount of exercise every week. Invariably, the number of people who raise their hand is always small.

Many people actually think that being diagnosed with diabetes or some other chronic health condition will be the thing that helps them maintain a regular exercise routine, because the consequences of not taking care of their health become so much more serious. However, as you probably know if you've read this far in this book, that is not always the case. In fact, having a potentially life-threatening disease makes some people *less* likely to take up a regular exercise program, because the temptation to try not to do anything to remind oneself of one's diabetes can be very powerful.

Exercise and Diabetes

As outlined above, exercise is generally a big help in managing your diabetes and preventing some of the related complications from occurring. Studies have shown positive effects on not only blood glucose but also on important factors related to blood pressure, triglycerides, good and bad cholesterol, and blood flow and circulation (Stewart 2002). Despite these findings, many patients worry that exercise will make their diabetes worse, rather than better. In the following section we will lay out what the recommendations are for gaining the benefits of exercise while minimizing the potential risks associated with exercise for people with diabetes.

Three Types of Exercise

There are three main types of exercise that are considered important for anybody wishing to integrate physical activity into their lives: 1) aerobic exercise, 2) strength training, and 3) increasing activity. Before initiating any of these types of increased physical activity, it's important to talk with your doctor about any complications or risks that you need to be aware of when establishing an exercise routine.

Aerobic Exercise

Aerobic exercise is any kind of exercise that brings your heart rate up continuously for a sustained period of time. This can be all kinds of different activities, such as brisk walking, running, biking, stair-climbing, swimming, or any kind of activity that makes you sweat. The current recommendation for aerobic exercise, whether diabetes is present or not, is at least thirty minutes per day, at least five days per week (Pate et al. 1995). This amount of exercise is related to the lowest risk of heart problems and the best overall effect on the body.

For most people who are currently not exercising at all, this does not mean that you should start exercising at as high an intensity as you can for thirty minutes a day, five days a week. Rather, you should work your way up to this goal if you're currently exercising little or not at all. In addition, there is some recent research (Mason et al. 2006) that shows that there are better effects for your body if you spread out your aerobic exercise throughout the week rather than trying to fit more in on one or two days. For instance, if you only have an hour a week to exercise, it's better to exercise for twenty minutes on three days than for one hour on one day.

Aerobic exercise has many benefits for your cardiovascular system and is a wonderful way to decrease blood pressure, increase blood flow, and reduce stress. However, aerobic exercise also carries a degree of risk for individuals with diabetes. We talk about these risks in more detail below, but it is especially important to talk with your doctor and make sure you're prepared before starting an aerobic exercise workout.

Strength Training

Another form of physical activity that is important for people with diabetes is strength training. This involves using resistance of some kind, whether it is weights, exercise bands, or cans of food from your cupboards, to build up the muscles in your body. Many times, when we talk with our patients about strength training, the first thing they imagine is a bodybuilder or a muscled weight lifter, and they usually tell us "no thanks." When we talk about strength training, though, we're not referring to bulking up. Rather, we are talking about training your muscles to be more efficient and stronger so that your body uses its own insulin more efficiently, when this is an issue, and burns more calories even when you aren't exercising.

It works like this: Your body burns a certain number of the calories you eat each day just on running power—sort of like the basic electricity you use in your house even if you don't run a lot of high-powered appliances. This base number of calories burned is based on your size, your activity level (if you are an active, semi-active, or sedentary person), and your body's own personal thermostat or metabolism. When you add muscle mass to your existing frame, those muscles require more energy to function properly. Thus, you are basically turning up your thermostat or running a very high-powered appliance in addition to your already running power needs. This increase in power needed means more calories are burned even when you're just sleeping or sitting on the couch, watching TV.

Just like with any type of exercise, people with diabetes have to take some extra precautions when it comes to strength training. First, it is always a good idea to talk with your doctor about any potential adjustments you may need to make before starting a strength training routine. People with high blood pressure, blood vessel complications, or eye problems may need to use special care.

Second, it is always a good idea to get help developing and implementing a strength training routine. For some people, this means hiring a personal trainer who has received extensive training on helping people establish a weight-lifting routine and who will understand the possible limitations present due to your diabetes. If this option is more than you can afford or if you prefer not to go this route and you belong to a gym, once you have discussed your limitations with your doctor you can often ask one of the gym employees to demonstrate each of the weight machines for you to help you understand how they are operated and what muscle groups they target. Or you can seek a demonstration from a friend, family member, or colleague who regularly lifts weights; often people are more than willing to show a new strength trainer the ropes.

One more safe method of weight training is to lift light weights very slowly, counting to eight while you slowly lift and release, with enough repetitions that your muscle feels exhausted for the last two or three of the repetitions. This is a neat approach because it is super easy to integrate this into your day if you don't mind looking a bit odd. For example, most of us can easily raise a gallon of milk while doing a single "curl" (and if a gallon is too much weight, use a quart instead). While shopping in the store, it's an easy matter to do several very slow curls with a gallon of milk in one hand while shopping with the other. You will be shocked how quickly your muscles are exhausted even though the weight is small, because the slow, extended motion does not allow the muscle to rest. This approach is often safer than regular weight lifting because a light weight puts less strain on your tendons and joints, has low risk of injury, and allows good form to be maintained throughout the exercise. The fact that the weight is light does not mean it won't do as much; we know that once the muscle is somewhat exhausted, the biological trigger to grow more muscle is pulled. Then you just need to let it rest for a day while the new muscle is built. You don't need large, heavy weights to do weight training.

Once you see this possibility, many parts of the day can be used for weight training. While standing in line, you can gradually go up on your toes several times; while taking out the trash, you can gradually raise small trash bags out to the side; while doing the dishes, you can very slowly do shallow knee bends. It can be quite fun to find clever ways to safely move your muscles slowly with weight on them until they are slightly exhausted. And the slight feeling of burning in those last two or three repetitions is a good time to practice mindfulness and acceptance, as you notice slightly uncomfortable feelings that come up as you move toward your values.

Whatever your method for introducing strength training into your regular workout, it is important to remember that, just like with any exercise, you should start slowly and work your way up to more challenging weights or repetitions. This will prevent you from taking on more than your body can handle and possibly setting your routine back with a painful injury. Also, remember that if your goal is to increase your overall metabolism and increase the efficiency of your body's use of insulin, it is important to target major muscle groups like leg muscles and abdominal muscles to maximize your body's ability to build large muscles and therefore burn more calories to feed them.

Increasing Activity

The last type of physical fitness that needs to be addressed in a chapter about exercise is the idea of increasing your daily activity level to maximize your overall fitness level. This is a little different from incorporating aerobic exercise or strength training routines into your weekly or daily schedule. Instead, the purpose here is to increase your overall activity level every day in order to obtain the benefits of bringing exercise into your plan without having to schedule an extra workout to accommodate it.

When we first start talking about increasing activity with patients, their first response is usually "Great! I'll do that instead of aerobic exercise or strength training!" Unfortunately, it doesn't usually work that way. It is important to raise your heart rate for an extended time period multiple times a week and to build muscle, and increasing your daily activity does not always accomplish these goals. So, unless the extra activity you get is raising your heart rate and making you sweat or building the major muscle groups in your body, increasing the amount of physical activity you get every day should supplement a regular aerobic and strength building exercise routine, not replace it.

So what do we mean when we say "increasing activity"? It's simple, really. This entails literally taking extra steps every day to incorporate activity into your life. For example, you could try taking the stairs instead of the elevator, parking in the furthest parking spot and walking in to the office and back every day, and walking to the grocery store on Saturday rather than driving the few blocks in the car. These little things, and the dozens more that you could probably come up with very quickly, slowly add up to an increase in overall fitness, which leads to lower blood glucose and less weight.

One of the increasingly popular ways to keep track of activity during the day is by wearing a pedometer, which counts the number of steps taken. This doesn't give you all the information that would be necessary to determine the effects of the increased activity on your fitness, like your heart rate and the amount of muscle built, but it does give you an overall picture of how active you have been for the day. A typical goal for a person who would like to increase their fitness and/or lose weight is to take up to ten thousand steps per day.

This is no easy task, and we have to say that most of the time when people are meeting this goal, they are getting aerobic exercise as well, since it's hard to take that many steps during the day without your heart rate going up! A goal of ten thousand steps is often what people are aiming for, but that doesn't mean they start there; a goal of five thousand or eight thousand steps to begin with is a good way to start to see the benefits of increasing your activity level.

A good example of how incorporating more activity can lead to positive outcomes can be observed in the case of Carl. Carl is a forty-five-year-old man who had been diagnosed with diabetes five years before coming into our clinic. He was referred to us because his glucose levels were out of control, and he was having difficulty bringing them down. When we talked with Carl about the benefits of exercise, he stated that he did not think we should waste our time: he was never going to exercise, and we were not going to convince him to do it no matter what we said. Then, one of our colleagues suggested that instead of talking about exercise with Carl, we instead talk about activity. When we tried this, he was much more open about discussing the idea, so we forged ahead.

We told him not to think about it as exercise but rather to think about adding a little bit more activity to his day every day and to see how that impacted things. He agreed to give it a shot, and we asked him to come back in a month and tell us how it was going. A month later we couldn't believe the changes. First off, Carl told us that he had been able to increase his activity so much that when we added it up, we realized that he was now getting about forty-five minutes of aerobic exercise a day, just by riding his bike to the train station and walking up and down the stairs at work instead of taking the elevator. He told us that he had started taking extra trips downstairs in his office building when he needed a break from working, and that he had noticed that with very little effort he had lost about five pounds since we had seen him last. In addition, he stated that he had begun noticing that his blood sugars were consistently down in the target range, and he was hoping to talk with his doctor about reducing his medication soon. However, the nicest outcome, in our view, was that by the second time he came in to see us, he was interested in talking about adding consistent aerobic exercise and strength training to his routine. He was optimistic for the first time in years that he could achieve a level of fitness he had long since given up on.

The reason we were hopeful about Carl's case was that we knew that in order to help him meet his physical fitness goals, he would need not only to consistently elevate his heart rate every day and build muscle with aerobic activity and strength training, but also to do it in ways that were flexible, fun, and useful for him. Thus, increasing his overall level of physical activity served as a way for him to develop an exercise and fitness routine without forcing him to go to a gym or find an exercise class, since these were options he was not interested in.

Barriers to Exercise

When it comes to exercise, it seems there are always more reasons not to do it than to do it, no matter how much we talk about the benefits. When it comes to people with diabetes, the list of reasons for not exercising seems longer than ever. Below are some of the common reasons we hear for why our patients can't exercise. See if any of them sound familiar, if you are having a hard time with consistent exercise.

"I'm Afraid of What Will Happen to My Glucose Levels"

One of the biggest reasons people tell us that they are not exercising as regularly as they should is that they are unsure about the effect of exercise on their diabetes. If you have not had diabetes for long, you may fear the effects of exercise on blood glucose—particularly becoming hypoglycemic. This fear is often rooted in fact; excessive exercise can reduce blood sugar levels, and this is always something to watch out and be prepared for. However, given the overwhelming benefits of exercise and the ability to control the risks that are present, this barrier need not impact your ability to include exercise in your daily life, assuming it is okayed by your doctor.

"Exercising Hurts"

Not many people would willingly take part in an activity that caused pain every time they did it, especially if they weren't sure it would be helpful or at least less painful in the long run. Yet this is exactly the case for some individuals with diabetes when it comes to exercise. Whether it's neuropathy or circulation-related foot damage, there are many diabetes ailments that can make exercising more challenging. Harold, a sixty-one-year-old man whose diabetes had been very out of control for a long time, told us that exercising was something that would never be part of his life due to painful neuropathy in his feet and legs. He said that the medication he was prescribed did not help much with the pain, and he spent most of his waking life feeling as though his feet were being burned. Because of this pain, he had had to retire early and had not exercised for many years. He told us that he mostly stayed home and watched TV during the day, because it was painful to walk and he felt uncomfortable traveling around in a wheelchair. Given this pattern, it was not surprising that Harold had gained a considerable amount of weight and was constantly fighting to keep his blood glucose levels under control.

When Harold told us his story, we felt a little stuck at first. It was clear that he was in a tremendous amount of pain, and we did not want him to feel that we did not believe in his pain, or that we didn't think it was that big of a deal. At the same time, for us to agree with him that there was nothing that he could do but have a pain-filled life consisting of lonely TV-watching wouldn't help him live a meaningful life with diabetes. Thus, we spent the first part of our time with Harold letting him know that we could understand how overwhelming it must feel to be in his position and how other options for bringing activity and meaning into his life would seem impossible to think of from the position he was in. Then we explained that this is what he had hired us for—to be the problem solvers that find a way to bring these things into his life, even with all of the limitations he was facing.

We emphasized that while we thought his reasons were incredibly valid, that they were just that: reasons. And while reasons were useful in helping us make sense of why we did and didn't do things, they didn't really cause any behavior. For instance, in Harold's case, he believed that the *reason* he was not exercising was because he had too much pain. While it was true that he had a lot of pain and that there were many types of exercise he couldn't do, his having pain did not *cause* him to not exercise—his *believing* that he couldn't exercise with the pain did. When we encouraged him to investigate what happened when he noticed the thought that his pain made it impossible for him to exercise, rather than believing it, Harold quickly found that there were types of exercise that he could do, such as swimming and chair aerobics, and that he actually enjoyed them. His pain did not have to change for him to try these new ways of exercising; his belief that his pain was causing him not to be able to exercise did.

"It's Too Hot/Cold/Rainy Outside for Me to Exercise"

Another reason we often hear is that the weather outside is not conducive to taking a walk after dinner or a power walk at lunchtime. This reason is often given by people who inform us that walking is the only form of exercise they can tolerate, and when the weather is not good enough for walking, it's impossible for them to exercise at all.

One example of a person who had this belief was Ted, a fifty-five-year-old man with cardiovascular complications from diabetes whose diabetes and heart doctors were all encouraging him to take better care of himself with diet and exercise. At his first appointment with us, he informed us that he would only walk for exercise and that he wouldn't walk in the rain under any circumstances. Of course, when he made this statement, it was the beginning of the rainy season, which can last months in our part of the world.

When Ted informed us of these reasons, we asked him how believable, on a scale of 0 to 100, the statement that he would not walk in the rain was. He was very sure of himself and his contention against rain walking, so he told us it was a 100. We then asked him why he was coming to our clinic. He told us that he had been sent there to get help in better managing his heart disease and diabetes.

We then asked him why he would want to do that. He was clearly confused by the question and stated that he wanted to improve his health. So we asked him if he thought he would be able to do things to improve his health even if it meant doing things that were difficult or things he didn't feel like doing. He said that of course he would still be able to do those things, and that he knew that it would take work to get his health back under control. We then asked him why he would be able to do them. Again, confused by the question, he said because he wanted to live a long life. Again, we asked him why. He told us that he wanted to live a long life in order to continue to see his grandchildren, whom he had a very special bond with, grow up. So we said, "What if, in order to see your grandchildren grow up, you have to walk in the rain?" He thought about it for a minute and then said that he thought he would need to get an umbrella. Then we asked him again how believable on a scale of 0 to 100 his belief that he would not walk in the rain was. He did not even pause before saying "about a 10."

"I Have Tried to Establish an Exercise Routine Before and Failed"

Many people that we see in our clinic, and maybe some of you reading this book, have had the experience of trying to take care of their health and their diabetes and not being successful. For many, this has happened so many times that you feel as though you are powerless to ever make a lasting change. Thus, one of the biggest reasons folks with this experience have for not being able to exercise is the overwhelming thought that they just can't try and fail again. They become frustrated and find that things are much easier if they just give up trying and let themselves off the hook for a while.

This strategy makes a lot of sense. Not putting yourself out there, not trying again, is actually a very effective way to prevent having to feel things like disappointment, frustration, embarrassment, and sadness about the inability to take care of your diabetes and your health. In fact, we would say that this strategy is about 98 percent effective in helping keep these feelings far enough away to not have to feel them all the time (only 98 percent because in our experience, no matter how hard you try to keep these things down, a little always slips through).

The problem with this strategy, though, is that it requires you to live your life trying to move away from thoughts and feelings rather than toward your values and goals. It's as though you are the bus driver again at an intersection, and you must choose whether to turn right or left. To the right, you can (mostly) avoid feeling frustrated or disappointed in yourself for not meeting your own expectations. The only cost is that you have to go backward in your life.

To the left of the intersection, you can move forward in your life, toward the direction of your values and goals. The cost is that sometimes you will have to have thoughts and feelings you don't want to have, like disappointment and frustration when you try something and don't succeed. When patients tell us that the reason they can't exercise is that they don't want to fail again, they are telling us that they are at this intersection and are choosing to go right because it feels safer and easier. Again, it is their *belief* that this reason is causing their behavior that we want to look at; if that reason could be there and not stop them from heading left (because that direction is toward what they value), then heading left, toward exercise, would only become easier with time.

Getting Started

Before finishing up our discussion about exercise, it is important to talk about the necessary steps to take when beginning to exercise. The reality is that there are things that need to be taken into consideration in making sure your diabetes does not keep you from a regular exercise routine.

Talk to Your Doctor

As mentioned above, the first thing you must do before beginning any regular exercise is to talk to your doctor about any complications you have or are at risk for developing, and how they may impact the types of exercise you can choose from. Generally, individuals with very high blood pressure, eye problems, blood vessel problems, and nerve damage may need to choose types of exercise that minimize their risk of further complications or injury, and they may need to avoid lifting heavy weights. In addition, if you currently take oral diabetes medications or insulin, be sure to talk to your doctor about the best time to exercise in relation to taking these medicines and whether you should be looking out for signals that might indicate the need for a change in dose once your exercise routine becomes regular.

Make a Plan

Unlike a person without diabetes, there are a few things you need to prepare for before beginning an exercise routine. Planning in advance can help take any potential risks out of implementing an exercise routine and can make the process smoother, safer, and more enjoyable.

Identify Yourself

The first thing you need to do to prepare for an exercise program is to make sure that you have an ID bracelet that identifies you as a person with diabetes, in case anything were to happen to you while you are exercising. This precaution sometimes makes people feel uncomfortable with the idea of exercise; one patient told us, "You can stop right there. I changed my mind about exercising when the discussion started with how people were going to identify me when exercising made me pass out!"

While it's true that thinking about what will happen if you lose consciousness is not the most reassuring way to start preparations for starting an exercise program, it doesn't mean that you *will* lose consciousness because you are a person with diabetes who is exercising. It means only that it is possible for any of us to have an accident or take on too much while exercising, and if that should happen to you, it is important that people know that you have diabetes so they can determine the proper way to take care of you.

Snack and a Drink to Go

Another important element of exercising with diabetes is remembering to drink lots of fluids to avoid dehydration and to have glucose tablets, hard candies, or other quick sources of carbohydrate on hand in case hypoglycemia sets in. While these may not seem necessary for your workout, they are important to keep handy, because by the time you realize that you need them, it may be too late to track them down. In addition, your body needs extra fluid to work properly, given the action of diabetes on the body; so keeping an extra bottle of water on hand will help keep your system in tip-top shape for a workout.

Feed for Speed

While it is important to have glucose tablets or other forms of carbohydrate on hand in case of hypoglycemia, another important element in preventing low blood sugar problems is to have some food in your system well before initiating exercise. This is especially important if you are taking oral diabetes medications or insulin. Eating something one to two hours before starting exercise is ideal, although this is not always possible. If you don't have time to wait one or two hours after a meal to exercise, try having a small snack before beginning. In general, it's very important that you avoid skipping meals before you exercise.

Foot Patrol

The final element in preparing to become more active is to make sure you have a strategy for ensuring that you are taking good care of your feet. It's important to remember that foot complications are common in diabetes and are caused by relatively small cuts, scrapes, and injuries that don't heal normally given circulation problems present in many people with diabetes. The way to prevent a small foot problem from turning into a big foot problem is to remember to wear comfortable, cotton socks when exercising in order to minimize the risk of blisters or problems that result from excessive sweat and to wear comfortable, well-fitting shoes throughout your exercise routine. In addition, remember to check your feet after every exercise session to ensure that you catch any small problems early enough to take care of them.

Learn About Your Body's Response

Perhaps the most important thing to pay attention to in taking care of your diabetes as you initiate an exercise routine is your body's individual response to exercise, and how exercise affects your glucose levels. It can't be said often enough that everybody's body is different, and no two people—even two people with the same type of diabetes on the same medication—will respond the same to exercise.

To learn about your body's response, there are a number of steps you can take. First, check your blood glucose just before and directly following exercise. This will give you a sense of the immediate effects of that amount of exercise on your system. If possible, check your blood sugar again an hour or two later, since the glucose-lowering effects of exercise can extend out that long (this is important to remember in the prevention of hypoglycemia as well; don't put away those glucose tablets too quickly!).

If your blood glucose before exercise is below 100, have a small snack to prevent hypoglycemia. If your glucose is over 300 after eating or 250 fasting, wait until your levels have returned to below 250 or so before exercising to avoid the risk of it rising higher with exertion.

Also in terms of learning about your body, be sure that you pay attention to what the signs are for your body when it comes to hyperglycemia and hypoglycemia. Hypoglycemia is more common with exercise, but hyperglycemia can also occur if glucose levels are too high to begin with.

Hypoglycemia and Exercise

When watching for signs of hypoglycemia while exercising, you should pay attention to any changes in your heartbeat, increase in sweating, or feeling shaky, anxious, hungry, or dizzy. Obviously, it can be difficult to detect these while exercising in that some of these same symptoms (changes in heartbeat, sweating) are a normal part of exercising and do not necessarily indicate a problem.

When it comes to telling whether hyper- or hypoglycemia is present, the mantra we always tell our patients is "when in doubt, check" to determine if symptoms are due to blood glucose or are just a normal part of exercising. However, if you begin feeling shaky or dizzy, you should take a glucose tablet or drink a small glass of juice, in case these symptoms are due to hypoglycemia.

Hyperglycemia and Exercise

The symptoms of hyperglycemia, such as extreme thirst, fatigue, and frequent need for urination, are important to keep in mind when starting an exercise routine because if glucose levels are too high at the beginning of exercise, the exertion can sometimes cause glucose levels to temporarily spike. This can cause hyperglycemia, and again, some of the symptoms may mimic those of exercise, such as fatigue and thirst. As with hypoglycemia, it is important to check your blood glucose levels to see if the symptoms are due to exercise or if your glucose has risen too high.

Summing It Up

Exercise is one of the most effective things you can do to manage your diabetes and prevent many of the most dangerous complications.

Before beginning an exercise routine, make sure to talk with your doctor and take necessary precautions to minimize risks.

CHAPTER 9

Talking Diabetes

One of the goals of this book is to help you understand that you are not alone in coping with diabetes. Having said this, it can really feel like you are, especially when your friends, family, or other loved ones don't understand and can't talk to you about the highs and lows of diabetes self-management. Or, at least sometimes it seems that they can't talk to you in a way that you find helpful. This can make any of us feel alone. One of the best ways to deal with feeling isolated is (you guessed it) connecting to others. The way to connect is through communication. For us, that means "talking diabetes" with others.

The goals of this chapter are to talk about and teach you some basic skills that are directly related to acceptance, commitment, and coping with diabetes. Most of this book is really focusing on you and how you approach the successful management of this disease. This personal process is fundamental to living a values-based, healthy life. And, from a very practical perspective, we all have other people in our life we need to talk to. This can include doctors, nurses, friends, partners, spouses, children, relatives, teachers, and so on. We'd like to ensure that you have the skills to speak to others in a way that will allow you to get the most support you can, enabling you to talk about your feelings in an effort to help you both have your feelings and move in the direction of your values. The best place to start this discussion is to talk about why talking matters.

The Importance of Communication

So, talking matters—but why? Why can't those people who really know us, who really want to help us, just *know* what we need? They do this so well so often. In fact, we frequently rely on others to help us get our needs met and don't have to ask them directly to make this happen. If you are eating a salad, and a hungry friend says to you, "That looks good," then you will likely offer them a bite of your salad. In fact, you may offer to get them some salad of their own. If a friend calls and says "I feel sad," you are likely to ask "What's wrong?" This is how we help each other out when we need it. It is very natural and often very effective.

So why bother talking about this? Because sometimes the process of communication with others doesn't work this well. In fact, in the examples we just mentioned, the communication is only effective if both people understand the "rules" of a very complex social process. When people don't follow these so-called rules, things break down. When this happens, we must look again to our values—is this a relationship that is important to me? Is it important that I get my needs met here? If so, understanding and improving communication becomes key.

Unfortunately, we don't always know the rules of communication. And the situation gets trickier when the rules change without our realizing it. Or, even worse, there are times when there are no real rules for how to talk and communicate.

The general golden rule of doing unto others as you would have done to you is a good one. Still, most of us can think of an example where someone has broken that rule with us. We may even be able to think of an example where we have broken it with others. We generally teach children that they should be polite and respectful, and while these are good rules, they are not always followed. In fact, there are times, like in emergencies, that it is most expedient to disregard some of these rules, such as always being polite.

So, in this chapter on communication, what are we talking about? One of the most important purposes of communication is getting your needs met and meeting the needs of others. This can include giving and getting important information, giving and receiving help, talking about thoughts and feelings, and even sorting out differences. Again, how this relates to you in your life depends on your values for connection and relationships. This chapter will focus on giving you the communication tools to live in a way that is consistent with those values.

Styles and Strategies

How you say what you want to say is sometimes as important as what you say. Some people call this distinction *process* and *content*. The content is, of course, what you are actually saying, the meaning of the words you are trying to convey. The process is how you are communicating; that is, what is occurring while you communicate. Another way of talking about process can include our styles and strategies for communicating with others. These include how we use communication and how we go about getting our needs met.

In the examples above, giving someone some salad because they said that it looked good or helping someone out when they said they felt sad resulted when one of the speakers made a very particular type of request. This style of getting one's needs met could be called *passive* or *indirect*. Being passive or indirect is not necessarily a bad thing, certainly not always. Sometimes we equate passivity with negative things like passive aggression or being meek and helpless. In fact, much of our communication includes passive or indirect communication. When this gets us what we need and we are able to help others receive what they are indirectly requesting and the relationship feels positive, then there are often no issues with indirect or passive communication styles.

The Problem with Indirect Communication

The challenge, as you might predict, is that indirect communication is not always effective at helping us get what we need. It can require the person to whom we are speaking to interpret or guess what we're after. Not everyone is very skilled at making this type of guess.

After all, not many of us are mind readers. Still, those people we know, that we truly care about, that we have relationships with, can't they do this for us? The answer is, of course, yes—but not *always*.

One of the times that people can't guess what we need is when they don't understand what we are going through. Indirect communications can be very ineffective at getting others' support or help when they have no idea what we need support or help with. This is especially the case for a person with diabetes.

There is a very good chance that some of the material in this book is new to you. And you are the one that has been diagnosed with diabetes. Some of this information is complex and difficult to understand. The material here is directly related to *you* and *your* plan for self-management in a way that is not always easy to understand. Those people without a diagnosis of diabetes probably won't have all of this information. They may want to help, they may be very good at helping and supporting you in other ways, but they might not get this diabetes stuff at all.

The Difference with Diabetes

It's great that you've been able to get what you want or need from those around you just by dropping hints or communicating in this very natural and indirect way. But when you need to communicate about your diabetes with someone who hasn't got the disease, using the indirect approach may not work. They probably won't automatically know what you need or how your life has changed with your diagnosis, and they may not readily meet your needs. This disconnect might leave you feeling isolated and alone, especially if connecting with people in more direct ways is unfamiliar or unnatural.

For example, you now know that eating foods too high in sugar, fat, and carbohydrates can be very risky to your health. Even though it may not be apparent on the outside, these foods can be quietly damaging your blood vessels, heart, and nerves. So, you know to avoid these. But the people around you may not understand this right away. These folks love their food. *You* can love your food, but you have to make changes and choices and substitutions. If someone offers you a big bowl of delicious chocolate ice cream, that might seem insensitive or even mean. "How could they do that to me?" you might ask. We need a way to talk about this. Not only that, but if you ask for a big bowl of delicious chocolate ice cream, you need people in your life to know why this is not such a great idea. You need a way to have them understand how they can support you in that moment.

It doesn't end there, of course. As we have talked about repeatedly in this book, you have a lot of very natural, very difficult feelings that come up about your diabetes. These feelings include fear, anger, resentment, sadness, anxiety, and, well, too many to list. Talking effectively about these emotional experiences is very important. And it's hard for many of us to talk about these feelings. It's even difficult for others to hear about these feelings sometimes. We will get back to talking about feelings in just a moment, but right now let's focus on how to talk or communicate more effectively.

Effective Communication

So how can you communicate more effectively? We are positive that you are one step ahead of us on this. If talking about feelings indirectly or passively is not always effective, then the solution may be—you guessed it—being more direct in our communication with others. This is a lot easier said than done. And it can take practice to get good at it. A lot of practice. But try to remember that all of us, no matter how young, how old, how experienced, or how green, can learn new skills for communication. This can be difficult, but it's all for a good cause—helping you successfully manage your diabetes.

Assertiveness 101

One example of effectively communicating is making direct requests. This is often called being *assertive*. Now, we need to be really clear here that we are not talking about being aggressive. Being aggressive means that you are not taking others' feelings or needs into consideration and you are boldly just getting your own needs met, regardless of how others are impacted by your actions.

Being assertive means you are attempting to get your needs met *and* noticing that other people have needs, too. There are many things you need in life, and now, as you effectively manage your diabetes, there are likely more specific things you need—assistance, support, and so on—that are related to living a healthy and long life. The basic formula for asserting your needs looks like this:

When _____ happens, I feel (or think) _____. I understand that you might feel/need _____.
I would like _____ to happen instead. Can you help me with this?

This is very simplistic, and yet it is surprisingly effective at helping people assert what they need. You might notice that this very statement has some of the qualities we have been encouraging throughout—it is accepting, mindful, and values-based, for example. You don't need to use the exact words we've suggested, but if they help, try that. The blanks are for you to fill in with whatever you need or want in your interaction with another person. Remember that there are many, many ways to get your needs met. Even with direct communication, you can try this many different ways, using many different types of wording, and still get what you need. The real art of this process is to find how it best works for you.

Assertiveness in Action

To understand this concept, imagine that you meet your best friend, a real connoisseur of fried and fatty food, for lunch once a week. The problem is that he always picks restaurants that serve notoriously unhealthy food choices. Maybe you haven't wanted him to feel bad about his choices, or you haven't wanted to talk about your diabetes, so you haven't said anything. Or maybe until you read this book, you were still trying to avoid thinking about this whole diabetes thing, so you've just gone along with his choice of restaurants.

So now here you are, at another super-fat food emporium, trying to figure out how you are going to live your value of managing your diabetes in order to have a healthy life. You feel bad, and you wish you weren't here. You're stuck. What would an assertive, direct request look like? Remember that there are many ways to try to accomplish this. What if you tried this?

"You know, I am not sure how to say this, but I want you to know something. When you *choose fast-food restaurants*, I feel *really stuck and like I can't make healthy choices for myself*. I understand that you *enjoy the food, and it does look really good. And I know you're not trying to make me feel stuck at all*. I would like *for us to make picking the place we go to eat part of the fun of going out to lunch together, and I need to have a few more options for food*. Can you help me with this?"

The underlined parts in italics here are basically the blanks filled in from the example above. Notice that we changed the wording a little bit because that is closer to our style of talking. Still, we followed the basic formula. It's quite a mouthful, we know. However, the communication here is very clear. You are trying to have the other person understand your position without putting them on the defensive. You know they are not doing this to you on purpose, and in fact, they may feel bad that they didn't know that this was going on. You are also trying to enlist their help by asking "Can you help me with this?"

Shaking Up the System

Other people may not be used to you making direct requests. This can shake up a personal or family system that has evolved with your style and their style of communication. You need to be prepared for not always getting what you ask for, even when you do an amazing job of asserting yourself. Remember, too, that just like with humor, timing is everything. There are times and situations that may make it more likely for you to get your needs met. Try different ways of asking and in different situations to see if you aren't more successful.

Backing Off Being Assertive

But maybe you don't see yourself as having a problem with directness. Maybe you're even quietly giggling to yourself, thinking, "Oh, people *wish* I was more passive and indirect." But you still notice that you're not always getting your needs met, feeling listened to, or receiving the support you need. Well, remember that communication is a two-way street. The challenge with being too direct lies with others feeling that they don't count in the interaction. The golden rule and being polite and respectful are central here. It's very important to remember that other people have needs and feelings, even if it doesn't always seem that way.

When making requests related to successfully managing your diabetes, remember that demands ("you have to do this") or ultimatums ("do this, or else") usually don't go very far toward getting your needs met—especially when others don't understand why you are making such demands. While it's not unreasonable to want to tell someone, "Get that slice of cheesecake away from me!" they may not understand why. As we've said before, diabetes, while surprisingly common in our culture and on the rise, still remains a mystery to many people. They may think, "What would one little slice of cake do? Why do you have to be that way?"

What we want to do in our effective communication is to help people understand that it isn't just the one piece of cake; it is part of a series of decisions you are trying to make in order to live your values. But other people aren't always going to understand this. We need to help them understand. And this is where practicing positive, effective, direct (and respectful) assertion is so important.

Feeling Stuck

You may be saying, "This is all very good, but I just get so upset when I need to do this that I really can't assert my needs at all. It's just too hard." We understand. We really do. This *is* hard—*and* we need to keep making those choices that are best for living a healthy life.

Talking About Feelings

One of the key concepts of this book is that you can have difficult thoughts and feelings. They are our experiences. You can have absolutely overwhelming thoughts and feelings and still move forward in your life. And in this case, you can have them and still communicate what you need to the people in your life.

Often when talking to others about your experiences, the very emotion that feels so hard, that feeling you don't want to share, *that* is the thing that's really important to have other people understand. It is very important to communicate important feelings to other people.

Talking about your feelings can be very difficult. You might ask: "Where do I start?" "What is the best way to say what I feel?" "What if I don't even know what or how I feel?" All of these are perfectly reasonable questions to be asking yourself. They can also seem like really great reasons not to talk to others about our feelings. But wait—you're not off the hook so easily. While they *seem* like good reasons to avoid talking to others about our feelings, the reality is that they're not. They can be scary thoughts, but they don't have to stand in the way of you getting what you need.

"I Don't Know Where to Start"

That's easy. Just start anywhere. The person you are talking to about your feelings may be a little confused, just like you would be. But you can help them to figure this out. In fact, you can help each other make sense of all of this by simply beginning to talk. As you've probably heard before, just begin at the beginning. Start where you think it makes sense to begin trying to convey what you would like. If you don't know where that is, just jump right in.

"What Is the Best Way to Say What I Feel?"

There are no right or wrong feelings, and there are certainly no right and wrong ways to talk about them. There are certain things that are often helpful to keep in mind, like taking ownership of your feelings rather than blaming the other person for the way you're feeling. This issue will be addressed in just a little bit. Even still, there is no one way or even one best way to say what you feel. Remember that you are trying to help others help and understand you. Taking a breath, knowing that this is challenging, and letting others be there to help in this process is a great way to begin communicating your feelings.

"I Don't Even Know What I Feel"

Join the club (and it's a very big club). Almost all people at some time don't know what they feel—they just feel something. Putting a name to it can be very challenging and can often feel inadequate. *That* you are feeling something is the most important thing to keep in mind. Whether you name it correctly is really not the issue.

When someone asks "What's wrong?" and you come back to them with "Nothing," that makes it hard for them to respond. You may even be giving the wrong message. That is, you may be saying to them "Leave me alone" without realizing it. It's certainly okay to need your own space, but it might be more effective if you clearly request that from the other person. (You might try, "I need a little space" rather than "Leave me alone.")

On the other hand, if you would like to talk and just don't know how, that's another issue. One of the best things you can say is "You know, I don't know what I feel, but I sure could use someone to talk to." The other person isn't going to necessarily know exactly what to say, but they will know you want to talk.

Think about the variety of feelings you could be having right now. You could be frustrated. Thinking about all of this diabetes information is hard. You could be tired of doing fingersticks and having diabetes. You could be scared ("What if I lose my vision?"). You could be angry ("Why did I get stuck with diabetes!"). You could be sad

("Having diabetes makes me feel hopeless"). You could feel optimistic ("I *can* take good care of myself!"). And you know what? You could be all of these things at once. That's a lot to communicate.

Taking Ownership of Your Feelings and Thoughts

One thing we want to emphasize in both assertion and in talking about your feelings and thoughts is owning your own experiences and not making others responsible for how you feel or think. We often hear people say, "You made me feel _____ (fill in the blank)." While it is absolutely true that others can say things or do things that cause us to feel a variety of responses, it is rarely effective to blame them for our reactions. *We* feel our feelings. *We* think our thoughts. Telling someone else that they made us feel or think something puts them on the defensive, and we are less likely to have an effective or productive discussion. Instead, you might try saying that when something happens, *you* feel a certain way. This will help the other person understand the impact of their actions without putting them on the defensive, allowing for a better connection so that you can get your needs met and live your values.

Getting Everyone Else On Board

Remember that others without diabetes (and even some of those people with diabetes) don't always understand what you are going through. But they can! And you can help by conveying your feelings. On paper, another person can read that you need to change your diet, exercise, and do all the things you need to do to keep your glucose in control. But what does that really mean to them? This information would be read on the page just as instructions on complicated car repair would be read by most people—it wouldn't mean much and wouldn't keep their interest very long. It's okay if some people hearing about your diabetes are not terribly interested, because it does not directly relate to them. But for *you*, it reads very differently. It is important, it is vital, it is scary. It is frustrating, it is sad, it is optimistic—it is everything that you feel. Naturally!

Your job is to convey to others what you feel and what you need. They may never fully understand the facts and details that are so much a part of your life now, but we promise they can understand your feelings. Understanding your feelings will help them be on your side as you manage your diabetes.

The timing and situation you choose to discuss your feelings can also be important. Not every situation will meet with an open response from the person you're talking to. In fact, there are some situations, like being on a crowded bus, during a business meeting or religious service, or riding an elevator, where talking about your true feelings may be more difficult for you to do and may be difficult for others to respond to you. That makes sense. There are other situations that will make this easier. Sometimes it depends on the person you are talking to and sometimes it depends on you.

The fact that you need to be thoughtful about when and where you talk doesn't get you off the hook of talking to others about your feelings. In fact, you will likely find that it really helps others to understand your difficulties. This is especially important when enlisting others' support in your plan for managing your diabetes.

Relating This Back to Your Plan

The whole reason we are spending so much time on communication is that we want you to enlist the support of others in making your plan for successfully managing your diabetes more effective. Without the help of people in your life, the task of managing your diabetes—already very difficult—becomes that much harder because you are doing it all alone.

Remember Your Values and Your Loved Ones

A large focus of this book has been on helping you define what your values are and how they relate to taking care of your diabetes and your feelings about doing that. You know what you want in your life. And, if you are still reading, you value successfully managing your diabetes to live a long, healthy life.

The important people in your life—your doctor, your nurses and health care providers, your family, your friends, and your coworkers—they want this for you, too. Remember though, that they don't always understand how to best help you. Talking about your feelings, thoughts, and values and making clear requests can really help with this.

In the face of your feelings, *with* your feelings, you can let other people know what you feel, what you need, what you care about, and how they can help you. With friends and family, you may even have to educate them on just what this whole "diabetes thing" is all about (we will talk a little more about this later). Talking about what you need and how this makes you feel will really help them under-stand diabetes and your strategies for self-management, and talking can enlist their support in this process. You can, of course, go it alone and try to do all of this yourself. But you may discover that this path can be very difficult; and what's more, those close to you will feel left out of this important part of your life. You may find they are really ready to help and be there for you, but again, they might not know exactly how. That's where you come in with these skills as you live your values.

Remembering to Make Room for Others

So here is the bottom line: all of the difficulties you are having, well, you are absolutely not alone. Other people have them too. Just like you, others want to avoid talking about what they feel. They don't want to talk when you ask, "What's wrong?" They actually get anxious about your diabetes and then they can do the strangest things.

This book is not long enough to list all of the goofy things that people we care about do when trying to help us manage our diabetes. Everyone reading this book has a unique person in their life who has done something odd when confronted with you living with and managing your diabetes. Everyone. Here are just a few of the types of reactions you may have already encountered in your efforts to take care of your diabetes.

The Total Avoider

This is the person who, when you talk about your diabetes, try to educate them a little, or even share your feelings with them, won't have any of it. They are tough to deal with, for sure. You might get an enthusiastic "You're fine!" or even "Nah, you look great!" or even "I never trust what those doctors say." You may even get a few strange looks when reading this book. "Why do you have to spend so much time on this diabetes stuff?" or "Give it a rest, would you?" Not too supportive, huh?

The Freak-Outer

In some ways these people are on the opposite end of the continuum from the Total Avoiders. Your feelings and information about your diabetes are just too overwhelming for them. They feel their own natural feelings, but they feel them very strongly and very much out loud. It's a good thing for them to share their feelings, but their manner of doing so may actually increase your responsibility as you find yourself trying to calm them down. If you are spending all of your time soothing others, it may become difficult to also get *your* needs met. In fact, you may find yourself not sharing much about your diabetes with these people at all. That's where we get into trouble with this group.

The Bossy-Bosser

These are the people who take it upon themselves to bark orders, tell you what to do, what to eat, when to exercise, and otherwise take control and totally arrange your life. They become not just the boss, but the bossiest boss ever. You can't get a word in edgewise with these folks, and even when you can, they still know best. Again, that's a bit of a problem.

The Babier

For this last group, you are going to get a combination of some of the types above. They are worried about you, which is nice; but the way it is conveyed is just plain annoying. Suddenly you are the little baby again, and you need to be taken care of. Now, this is sweet, but the way it comes across is sort of like the Bossy-Bosser, and you no longer have choices about what you do or how you do it. *They* know what is best. Which means, in this situation, *you* don't. Do you see a problem?

Making Room for Others' Reactions

The bottom line for all of these types is that people are communicating with you in a way that doesn't work well. Responding in these ways doesn't help you to successfully manage your diabetes and may even be pushing them away from you. Though this may feel very frustrating, try to keep in mind that these people are doing the best that they can, given what they know and what life has taught them so far. Even though they are doing their best, you can help them do a little better, given what you need in that interaction.

And, the reality is, they are scared for you. This is just how they're showing it. This is their version of communicating their feelings. You have a disease that they may or may not understand. Typically, they don't know that you have a great deal of control you can exert over the disease, even though you know this. They are angry that this has happened to you. They are frustrated that they may have to make changes. They may be annoyed that they are out of control of your health (even though they were never in control). They are confused. They have every emotion and thought that you can think of. The reason they feel all of this is that they care about you and are invested in your health—even if they don't seem like it from their behavior.

Just like when you weren't sure how to talk about your feelings, they don't know how to respond to theirs. You are learning some fine tricks, some strategies and styles, for communicating with others. They don't have these yet.

Still, responses like these can set up conflict with these important people. But don't worry, conflict just means you are temporarily stuck in a holding pattern of communication. There are plenty of ways to break out of this pattern of interaction.

Effectively Resolving Conflict

One of the best tips that we can offer concerning communication is that it's often easiest to get the support and assistance from others when you make the problem a group problem. "Can you help me?" or "Can we work on this?" is very different from "Do this better. Now!" Remember that you're not trying to have the other person feel like they are doing something wrong, if they are not really aware that they are. You can help them understand that whatever they are doing just isn't working very well, but that the two of you can absolutely do things differently. Together.

All of the four types of responses we listed above have the common factor that they reflect care about you. People responding in these ways want to help you, and they want to be there for you. They just don't know how to do this effectively yet. Remember your values here. Where do relationships fit with your values? Where does getting help and connecting with others fit into your plan for successfully managing your diabetes? This is the place from which to start when addressing conflict or making requests from others about engaging you and this process differently.

As an example, to the Total Avoider you could say: "I know you are scared and confused by this." (Don't expect the Total Avoider to admit to these feelings just yet.) "I'm scared, too. This is a scary process for both of us. It has taken me a while to even feel like I could talk to you about this. But, it is important for you to understand what I'm going through and what I need to successfully manage my diabetes and live a long, healthy life. I want to understand how this is affecting you, too. You are very important to me, and you are very important in helping me manage this disease. It's okay if you don't want to talk about things now or even tomorrow, but I want you to know how I feel and what I need. Can you do that with me?"

As another example, you could tell the Babier how much you appreciate their concern, but that it really feels like too much. This might sound something like this: "I really like that you care so much about me. But the way it shows up in our relationship, like when you say that I can't have certain things or when you take food off of my plate, feels like you think I'm incompetent. I know that you don't mean for me to feel that way, and I need you to try something different here. Instead of taking away my choices and options without asking me first or assuming that I don't know what is best, can you ask me how I feel about it? I think that would really help me. What are your thoughts about this?"

Always remember that your voice, your style, will be different from theirs. There is no one right way to do this. Your goal, consistent with your values, is to help this person understand what you need and how you feel. You will likely have to come at this from a lot of different angles. It will be worth it for you to keep trying, though. Their reaction is a strong one, and at its core is a strong sense of caring for you.

Educating Others

A big part of this chapter is really telling others, even teaching others, what will help you become and stay effective at managing your diabetes. Part of teaching others is making sure you understand what you need to know about diabetes. One thing you might hear a teacher say to a student is "If you can effectively explain this to someone else, then you know the material." What these teachers are trying to convey is that it's one thing to read material or hear it told to us but is quite another to find a way to put that information into your own words and share it with someone else.

You have read several times in this chapter that our job is to get others on board with our plan for diabetes self-management. It is very helpful to practice putting this information into your own words and communicating it to others. This strategy can be helpful with everyone from coworkers, to friends and family, to your doctor and health care providers.

Talking to Your Doctor and Other Care Providers

Your doctor and other health care providers know a great deal about diabetes. They can provide you with a lot of information about the disease. What's more important, though, is that they can help you understand the information we are trying to convey to you in this book in ways that may make even more sense to you, and they can help make sure your understanding of the facts about diabetes and self-management is completely accurate. It is important that you talk with your doctor, diabetes educator, nutritionist, or other health care provider if you don't fully understand some aspect of this information or other things you have heard about diabetes. They will help you become clearer about information that can directly affect your health.

Showing Off Your (Diabetes) Investment

Another reason it is so important to talk with your doctor and health care providers is to show them how invested you are in effectively managing your diabetes. You can convey this partly by sharing with them the knowledge you have about diabetes. These care providers can certainly correct any mistakes in the information you possess, but more importantly you will be showing them that you are not a passive person in your treatment. You are in charge and continue to be your best advocate in your diabetes management. By talking about your disease, its complications, and your medications, you are showing the health care providers you are as committed to your health as they are. In fact, you are the most committed.

This actually gives you both common ground and a common set of goals to work toward. If your health care provider has suggestions or advice to offer, you can listen and then provide thoughtful comments and questions. If they are bossy with you, you can say that you understand this information and ask them to help you implement the knowledge you already have or are coming to understand. If they baby you, you can let them know that you are taking this disease by the reigns and that you are playing an active role in your process. You want to be able to communicate with your doctor and health care providers that you understand the seriousness of your self-management, and that you are working hard to live a healthy life. This can have a big effect on your interactions with them and can make a positive impact on your life.

Summing It Up

Clear communication can help you get your needs met by friends, family, and health care providers.

Knowing your relationship values will help you determine what to say to loved ones about your diabetes; assertive communication skills will help you determine how to say it.

CHAPTER 10

Medication Meditation

Medication is an important part of good management for most people with both type 1 and type 2 diabetes. If you have type 1 diabetes, insulin is such an integral part of how your diabetes is controlled day to day that management without this addition is almost unimaginable. We will discuss insulin, how it works, and the considerations for taking it later in this chapter.

If you have type 2 diabetes, however, the use of medications and insulin may be a little more confusing. This is because when you were first diagnosed with having type 2 diabetes, depending on your blood glucose levels, medication may not have been prescribed immediately. Then, when and if it is prescribed, there are so many different options that seem to do very different things and have such different side effects that the decisions between medications might seem beyond comprehension. To make matters worse, for many people, if blood sugar levels decrease enough and diet and exercise improve enough, the same diabetes medications that seemed to be helping might be taken away. This can make the whole issue of taking medications difficult to understand and follow as prescribed.

You probably know that there are many, many drugs out there that get prescribed for a whole host of problems. You see ads in magazines and, in the last decade, you can see drugs advertised on television. What are they for? Who takes them? Do you have to take them? Are they safe? These are all questions that you may have asked yourself.

Medication Considerations

There are a number of factors that need to be weighed when considering the different types of medications out there and which will be best for you and your diabetes management. Contemplate these factors and then discuss them and the issues they bring up with your doctor to make sure that you're giving yourself the best possible chance for succeeding in your diabetes management.

Mechanism

One of the most important factors to consider when selecting among diabetes medications is the mechanism of the drug. What we mean by *mechanism* is the way that the drug works to lower overall blood sugar levels. Some medications work by impacting the amount of insulin produced in the body, while others work by targeting insulin resistance. This is an important aspect to pay attention to because if your body is resistant to insulin, it won't matter how much insulin is generated—your body will likely still not respond to it. The importance of this is well-illustrated with the experience of one patient of ours, Larry, a sixty-one-year-old man recently diagnosed with type 2 diabetes. Larry had many family members with type 2 diabetes, and a number of them had been helped with a class of drugs called thiazolidinediones (see discussion below), which directly target insulin resistance, or the inability of the body to use insulin effectively. Larry's body, however, was simply not producing enough insulin, and it was using what it was producing just fine.

When Larry found out that he needed to go on medication, he insisted to his doctor that he should take a thiazolidinedione drug, since these had been so effective for his relatives. His doctor tried to explain the different mechanisms at play, but Larry did not completely understand the difference and ultimately felt as though his doctor wasn't listening to him. Not surprisingly, he stopped taking the medication his doctor had prescribed and was eventually sent to see us to help get him back on track.

Fast-Acting or Long-Acting

Some medications are designed to mimic the short-acting effect of insulin in the body when food is eaten: they increase the availability of insulin quickly in order to deal with the glucose in the blood from that meal, and then they "shut off" to help the body return to normal. These fast-acting medications can start working as quickly as five minutes after they are taken. Longer-acting medications work to mimic the general buzz of insulin that is always present in the blood at low levels, which helps keep things from getting too high or too low between meals. Determining which of these formulas, or whether a combination of the two, is best for you is another factor to consider when selecting a drug regimen. Again, this selection is based on your body's needs; if you have an adequate amount of insulin most of the time but have a difficult time managing your blood glucose after a meal, a shorter-acting, more intensive formula might be more appropriate than one that boosts overall levels a small amount.

Single or Multiple Dose

One thing we know for sure is that nobody is 100 percent perfect at taking their medications 100 percent of the time. Thus, an important piece of the diabetes medication puzzle is determining the most realistic plan for you to succeed at your medication management. We will talk about both practical and psychological barriers to taking medications below, but one crucial element of selecting a medication or medications is to have an understanding of whether or not medications that must be taken multiple times a day are realistically something you can manage, or if a once-a-day regimen is more doable.

It's important to understand that by listing this as a consideration, we would still like you to note that your beliefs about whether or not you can or can't manage your daily medication regimen are still just that: beliefs. In other words, this is not to say that you could not manage to take your medications multiple times per day even if you didn't want to or didn't think you could, if doing so was consistent with your health values. Rather, we want to think about what will give you the highest likelihood of successful management considering your lifestyle.

To make this distinction, it is useful to look at two separate cases where taking medication was a significant problem. First, we consider the case of Richard, a forty-one-year-old attorney referred to us for help in managing his type 2 diabetes. Richard traveled frequently for work and told us that the biggest difficulty he had in keeping his diabetes under control was remembering to take his medications while he was traveling. He was on a regimen that required that he take medications multiple times a day, sometimes with food and sometimes without. With his busy schedule and the lack of consistency in his day-to-day life, he had a hard time keeping track of when he was supposed to take his medications and often took them at the wrong time and caused himself to become hypoglycemic.

While we definitely spent time talking with Richard about his values and what was most important to him in order to reprioritize diabetes care in his life, there were undeniably circumstances in his current work life that made it difficult to keep track of multiple doses of medication a day. When his doctor switched him to a longer-lasting regimen that he took only one time per day, his overall management improved dramatically.

Next, we consider the case of Ken. Ken was a sixty-five-year-old man with type 2 diabetes referred to us also because he was having a difficult time taking care of his diabetes. Ken was recently retired from the postal service and his control over his blood sugar had actually decreased since he had stopped working. When we first met with him, it seemed unusual to us and to Ken that now that he had more time to manage his diabetes, he wasn't doing as well at it as when he had more demands on his time.

When we dug a little deeper, however, we quickly found out that since his retirement began, Ken had been struggling with his mood. He'd been feeling a little disconnected and lonely, and he had begun spending large amounts of time on his couch watching television. Like Larry, Ken's medication regimen was reasonably complex, and in his current mood and state of mind, he often had the thought that he didn't have the concentration and energy to keep track of it all anymore.

Unlike Larry, Ken's problem was not a busy life that was making it difficult to keep his medications straight, but rather his belief that he couldn't manage it. Chances are, if Ken had been switched to a less complex regimen, it would also be too challenging or less important over time, given that it wasn't really the complexity that was keeping Ken from maintaining his management but his believing the thought that he could no longer do it.

Existing and Potential Complications

From heart disease to kidney damage, the type of drug you take to help control your diabetes has a big impact on complications or potential complications. One reason for this is the side effects of some medications. For instance, if weight gain and swelling are a side effect of a medication, it may not be the best choice for somebody who needs to lose weight or is at risk for heart disease or heart failure.

Additionally, the way the medication leaves the body is important to consider when choosing a drug. If the medication is excreted from the body through urine, this means that the by-products of the drug need to go through the kidneys. If you have kidney damage or kidney failure, this can be very hard on the functioning of your kidneys and can exacerbate existing problems. Conversely, if the drug leaves the body through feces, it means that it must go through the liver in order to be excreted. Again, if liver damage has occurred or is threatened, this type of drug should be avoided.

Side Effects

Side effects are another consideration when selecting a medication. With all different types of drugs, side effects are one of the most powerful determinants of whether or not the medication is taken as prescribed, because, well, people generally do not take medications that have terrible side effects.

There's no exception in the case of diabetes medications. If the side effect profile for a medication prescribed by your doctor is difficult to tolerate, it is important that you talk with him or her about switching medications in order to maximize the likelihood and the length of time you will take them.

There are other considerations in determining the right drug for you, whether they are financial or formulary constraints imposed by your insurer or economic situation, or effectiveness, or other factors that are more immediate in influencing the decision you and your doctor make about which medication or medications to take. But it is important to consider the entire picture when selecting the right diabetes drug for you. Below we describe in more detail how each of the different classes of drugs works, and we offer some information that may assist you in basing your choices and your discussion with your doctor on the considerations above.

Types of Oral Diabetes Medications

There are many types of diabetes medications out there, and for every class of drugs it seems there are an equal number of choices and decisions within each class. Luckily, there are dozens of books written about diabetes medications. Thus, we recommend that you use this information to educate yourself about the general functioning of each of the classes of medications for diabetes, as a starting point for discussions with your doctor, and in the pursuit of more information from more complete sources.

Sulfonylureas

Sulfonylureas are a very popular class of drugs that work by pumping up the action of the pancreas to make more insulin (see chapter 2 for a description of the role of insulin and glucose in the body). They also assist the body in utilizing existing insulin, which combines with the insulin-producing action to decrease blood glucose. The sulfonylureas are broken down into first generation and second generation drugs, with the first generation pills being generally milder than the second generation, meaning that they are less intense, and thus less likely to cause hypoglycemia. Hypoglycemia is an important consideration with this class, since they boost insulin in the body, which can lead to glucose levels falling too low. In addition to hypoglycemia, side effects of sulfonylureas include stomach irritation, skin rash or itching, and weight gain.

Generic Name	Brand Name
Glyburide	DiaBeta
Glimepiride	Amaryl
Chlorpropamide	Diabinese
Acetohexamide	Dymelor
Glipizide	Glucotrol, Glucotrol XL
Glyburide	Glynase PresTab, Micronase
Tolbutamide	Orinase
Tolazamide	Tolinase

Because there are many types of sulfonylureas, there is a range in terms of how quickly they work and how they should be taken. There are once-a-day formulations that are generally only taken before breakfast, and other types that are taken once before breakfast and once before dinner. Whichever type is taken, one further consideration with sulfonylureas is the failure rate. For some people, sulfonylureas are not effective from the start; for many others, they work initially but decrease in effectiveness after a few years. This means that even if this type of medication is effective initially, it will typically stop working within a few years, which can be frustrating.

Biguanides

Generic Name	Brand Name
Metformin	Glucophage
Metformin Hydrochloride Extended Release	Glucophage XR

Metformin, both the original formula and the extended-release version, have also become increasingly popular in recent years. One of the main reasons for this is the unique mechanism by which this drug works. Metformin actually intervenes in the liver to prevent too much blood glucose from being made, rather than increasing the amount of insulin your body generates to combat it. One consequence of this type of mechanism is that if taken alone, metformin does not increase your risk of hypoglycemia.

An unusual side effect of this mechanism for lowering blood glucose is that many people experience weight loss when they begin taking metformin. This is often a positive consequence for many people with type 2 diabetes, although the weight loss is sometimes due to stomach and gastrointestinal discomfort or a loss of taste for food. In addition to weight loss, metformin can also improve triglyceride and LDL (or bad) cholesterol levels, while increasing HDL (or good) cholesterol levels. Unfortunately, not all the potential side effects are this positive. Nausea, vomiting, and diarrhea can occur, as well as dizziness, fatigue, and difficulty breathing. In addition, people with kidney or liver problems should generally not take this drug, nor anybody who drinks more than two to four alcoholic beverages per week, or pregnant or nursing mothers. Metformin and metformin extended release should be stopped before surgery or any medical test that involves the use of a dye. Metformin is generally taken two to three times a day, with a meal, and the extended-release version is taken once a day, usually in the evening.

Alpha-Glucosidase Inhibitors

Generic Name	Brand Name
Miglitol	Glyset
Acarbose	Precose

Alpha-glucosidase inhibitors are designed to lower blood glucose by blocking the enzymes that break down more complex carbohydrates into what turns into blood glucose. Because of this mechanism, these medications must be taken with meals to be most effective and thus are recommended three times daily.

Also because of the way alpha-glucosidase inhibitors work, one unfortunate side effect is the generation of a high level of gastrointestinal discomfort: gas, abdominal pain, and diarrhea. There aren't many other common side effects, though, and hypoglycemia isn't caused by this class of drugs when taken by themselves. If they are taken with another drug, however, and hypoglycemia develops, it must be treated with glucose or more simple carbohydrates, since the alpha-glucosidase inhibitor will block the breakdown of more complex carbohydrates that go into the system and prevent blood sugars from returning to normal levels.

Thiazolidinediones (TZDs)

Generic Name	Brand Name
Pioglitazone	Actos
Rosiglitazone	Avandia

Thiazolidinediones, also known as TZDs or "glitazones," work by making the cells in your body more sensitive to the insulin that is present. In other words, this class of drugs specifically targets insulin resistance—a major problem for many people with type 2 diabetes.

Glitazones are somewhat unique among diabetes medications in that they are one of the only classes of drugs that take a long time to become really effective—it can be up to three months or more before you would start to see the drug's full effectiveness. In addition, once this medication is stopped, it takes a long time to clear the system. Clearance occurs through the liver, so this drug is not considered appropriate for people with liver problems, and an earlier type of medication in this class, troglitazone, was taken off the market in 2000 for causing serious liver problems. Newer drugs do not appear to have the same problem, but liver testing is done before the medication is started and periodically while it is being administered just to be on the safe side.

Other side effects can include swelling and weight gain, and this class of drugs has been shown to make birth control pills less effective. This is important to note, because drugs in this class can improve fertility as well, and women should not take this medication if they are pregnant or nursing. Thiazolidinediones are typically taken either once or twice daily.

Meglitinides/D-Phenylalanine Derivatives

Generic Name	Brand Name
Repaglinide	Prandin
Nateglinide	Starlix

Technically, *meglitinides* and *D-phenylalanine derivatives* are two separate classes of drugs, but their mechanism and profiles are similar, so we have grouped them together for our purposes here. These types of medications work by stimulating insulin production for the meal that directly follows their being taken. These drugs work fast and are out of the system within a few hours, so the risk of hypoglycemia is reduced, although still present.

One advantage to these fast-acting formulas is that although they are taken up to thirty minutes before every meal, if a meal is skipped, you do not take a dose of either of these medications. This means that you do not have to eat a meal if you're not hungry just so that you can take your medication. This may help with excess weight sometimes present in type 2 diabetes, although weight gain is a side effect of meglitinides, so the pros and cons of this type of medication should be considered carefully.

These medications should not be taken if you have liver disease, given that they are cleared through the liver, and care needs to be taken with certain types of kidney problems as well. Because they work in a similar fashion, these drugs should not be combined with sulfonylureas, but they are often combined with metformin.

Insulin

As we discussed in chapter 2, insulin is a hormone that is made by the body to regulate blood glucose. It is different from the oral medications described above, which are designed to help your body create more insulin or reduce blood glucose through other means, in that taking insulin literally means injecting ready-made insulin into your body to substitute for your body not making enough on its own.

For people with type 1 diabetes, insulin is a fact of life. From the time of initial diagnosis, insulin, and typically insulin injections, is part of the deal. For some, this is the worst part of diabetes management: keeping meticulous count of carbohydrates in order to give yourself an injection from one to many times a day.

For people with type 2 diabetes, the role of insulin is not as well defined. Many people with type 2 diabetes do not start out initially on insulin. If they do, they are usually put on it to give their bodies a rest from the toxicity that occurs in the pancreas cells from prolonged high blood sugar, and then they are taken back off the insulin and prescribed either diet and exercise or these with one (or more) of the oral diabetes medications discussed above. Over time, many people with type 2 diabetes may end up on insulin because other methods have failed to keep blood glucose levels down consistently. When this occurs, it often feels like a failure for the patient who is put on insulin, and we have seen many patients who feel frustrated and upset about having to take insulin. These people often have more difficulty maintaining control of their diabetes and taking their insulin properly, so it is worth a discussion about how insulin works here to clarify that being put on insulin is not a punishment for poor management: it is often a crucial piece of your overall diabetes management plan that will help prevent life-threatening complications from developing.

There are many different types of insulin, but unlike oral diabetes medications, all these different types have the same basic mechanism—they increase insulin in the body. Because insulin is a protein, which would be broken down by the body just like any other protein if taken orally, it must be administered directly into the bloodstream in order to be effective. As discussed in chapter 2, an increase in insulin in your body allows the blood glucose that is floating around in your bloodstream to enter into your cells and muscles. This gives your muscles the energy they need to function and reduces the amount of glucose potentially causing damage to nerves, organs, and tissue.

The different types of insulin available vary in the amount of time they take to start working, how long they take to lower blood glucose, and how long they work. These differences are important because, as mentioned above, your body has different levels of insulin working at a given time. For instance, when you wake up in the morning, a certain amount of insulin has been present overnight in your blood to work on the last meal you had the night before and to keep whatever glucose is in your blood moving into your cells. Then, when you have breakfast, your body creates a spike in insulin in order to deal with the load of glucose it just got from whatever food you just ate. This spike needs to be most effective during the time that the body is breaking down carbohydrates into glucose, and then it needs to turn off in order for your glucose levels not to drop too low and cause hypoglycemic symptoms.

Rapid-Acting Insulin (Insulin Lispro/ Humalog; Insulin Aspart/NovoLog)

Rapid-acting insulin, called Humalog and NovoLog by the pharmaceutical companies that market it, is considered a great advance in insulin and diabetes management because it allows you to take it right before eating and lowers the risk of hypoglycemia because it does not stay in the system as long as regular insulin (discussed below). Rapid-acting insulin begins working within as little as five minutes and lowers blood glucose levels within the first one to two hours. This type of insulin then stops working completely after about three to four hours, thus giving you a better chance of avoiding hypoglycemia altogether.

Short-Acting Insulin (Regular Insulin)

Before Humalog and NovoLog hit the scene, regular insulin was a mainstay for people taking insulin and was the choice to take before meals to try to combat the after-meal glucose spike. Regular insulin starts working in about thirty minutes and lowers glucose levels the most in about two to five hours. It takes about five to eight hours to completely leave the system, however, so the risk of hypoglycemia is higher, since the insulin is still present long after the after-meal spike has disappeared.

Intermediate-Acting Insulin (NPH or Lente Insulin)

Unlike rapid-acting and short-acting insulin, intermediate-acting insulin is not designed to mimic the insulin release that happens directly following a meal, but rather the steady state of insulin in the system all the time. This type of insulin begins working in one to three hours and lowers glucose for up to twelve hours. It leaves the system in about twenty-four hours.

Long-Acting Insulin (Ultralente Insulin)

Like intermediate-acting insulin, long-acting insulin is designed to keep smooth glucose control continuously for longer periods of time. This formulation begins working in four to six hours and keeps a low level of blood glucose control for up to twenty hours. It leaves the system after about twenty-four hours.

Very Long–Acting Insulin (Insulin Glargine/Lantus)

Very long–acting insulin is specially formulated to begin working quickly, typically within one to two hours, and keep a steady, low level of insulin in the bloodstream for twenty-four hours. Unlike other types of insulin, the steady rate delivered by insulin glargine does not peak during the twenty-four hours, and it does not matter what part of the body the injection is given in. It is usually taken once a day at bedtime, and it does not typically cause nighttime hypoglycemia, as some shorter-acting forms of insulin can do.

Premixed Insulin (NPH and Regular Insulin)

Although almost all of the above formulas can be mixed to create an insulin that targets both after-meal and basal-level (the amount the body needs throughout the day) insulin, a premixed formulation that combines regular and intermediate-acting insulin also exists. This allows you to have only one injection, while targeting both types of glucose control at once.

Barriers to Taking Diabetes Medications

As we discussed above, there are often many obstacles to taking diabetes medications and insulin when they are prescribed to you. Some of these barriers, like aversive side effects or complex regimens that are hard to follow, may be more practical or logistic barriers that can be addressed by talking with your doctor about switching medications or simplifying your pill-taking routine.

Other barriers, however, are less related to side effects or remembering and are more related to your thoughts and feelings about having diabetes and taking medications. This is an important, often neglected, part of improving your diabetes management. As we have discussed throughout this book, we often feel as though the way we think or feel about a certain issue determines how we behave. For example, if you have the thought that you cannot take your diabetes medicine because you don't feel like it, you may believe that because of this you actually *can't* take your medication.

A good example of this issue was seen with Sean, a thirty-nine-year-old man with type 1 diabetes. Sean was referred to us because he was having a hard time taking his insulin because he was afraid of injecting himself. He had tried other forms of insulin administration, such as pens and injection devices, but he continued to struggle, partly because he knew that he "couldn't do it," no matter what he tried. When he first came to see us, we asked him to list all of the thoughts he had about injecting himself. We found that his worry was not only about the pain of the injection, but also all of the anxiety he felt leading up to the needle going into his skin and the evaluations he had about himself for not being able to inject himself. All of these worries piled up on him every time he went to give himself his insulin. In addition, as time went on and he continued to believe that he was not able to inject himself, he began having vivid worries about what was happening to his body, given his out-of-control sugars, and all of these fears and worries also came up when he thought about injecting himself.

As you can imagine, after a while, Sean would do just about anything not to have to think about giving himself an injection, given all the negative thoughts and feelings he had to have when he even considered it. He stopped seeing his doctor and stopped talking about his fear with his friends and family so that they would assume it was going okay and not ask him about it. He only came to see us because his doctor had sent him a letter letting him know that she was worried. The doctor had made an appointment with Sean to see us; he had inadvertently left the letter in a place where his wife found it, and she made him come to the first appointment.

Once he had revealed all of his worries and fears to us, Sean reported feeling somewhat less overwhelmed by them, and after spending some time defining what his values were and practicing just noticing his thoughts and feelings rather than trying to eliminate them, he was able to bring all of his fears with him as he injected himself. He later told us that he began to think of the insulin as a kind of steroid that pumped up his "chessboard muscle," and that every time he injected himself he grew stronger in his ability to let his fears be there as he moved in the direction of his values.

Summing It Up

With medications and insulin, it is important to consider such factors as how, when, and how fast they work, as well as side effects and complication interactions, so that you have the best chance of taking them consistently.

Fears and worries about diabetes and thoughts about taking medication and insulin may feel like barriers to effective use.

CHAPTER 11

Preventing, Detecting, and Treating Complications

B y now, we have really told you most of what you need to know to successfully manage your diabetes and live a healthy life. There are a few more things to talk about, though, and this may be the most anxiety-producing part of having diabetes. Remember that in chapter 2 you were introduced to the concept of diabetes complications. That was not put in the book at that point to scare you. We know two things about scare tactics: 1) many times scare tactics get used by people to try to motivate someone to behave a certain way; and 2) scare tactics don't work.

Chapter 2 tried to introduce these concepts to you in a way that had you feel like you could understand what was at stake in managing your diabetes, it's true. And, you really need this information. What is most important, though, is that you understand that these complications are very, very preventable for most people. Diabetes is several things to people—scary, upsetting, and challenging—but it is not a disease with a predetermined outcome. In other words, having diabetes does not dictate your fate.

Using ACT

As we have emphasized repeatedly, complications of diabetes are difficult for everyone involved. No one wants to go blind, have heart disease, lose their feet, or die before they are ready. The tools given to you in this book are a huge part of the answer to successful self-management. The two biggest components for that success are learning to experience all of your thoughts and all of your feelings for what they are *and* committing to action that allows you to live your values. Having thoughts and feelings about losing your vision should scare just about anyone. Now, the question is, what do you do with those thoughts or feelings? Do they run wild? Are they so scary that you have to work your hardest not to think those thoughts or experience those feelings? Do they make you need to cope in unhealthy ways, like smoking or drinking alcohol, or eating to soothe your fears? Do you just want to avoid people and hide?

Now, of course, it is okay to have any of those thoughts and feelings. It's okay to want to run away, it is okay to want to drink or eat yourself into oblivion. The real trick to using the skills in this book, and we know you see this coming, is to have those feelings and do what you think is best for you. Are you moving in a valued direction when you smoke or drink? Is it consistent with your values of a healthy life to eat those foods that you know will raise your blood sugars, cause you to put on weight, and otherwise create more health problems? Are your goals to stay away from people and just avoid everything related to diabetes? You wouldn't be reading this book if the answer to these last questions was yes.

In that you are still reading this book, we know your goals are successful management of your diabetes. It is not only understandable to be afraid about diabetes complications, it is *perfectly natural*. All of your feelings are perfectly natural, remember that. Using acceptance and commitment therapy allows you to have these feelings and do what you need to do, what you want to do, to take care of your health. Remember these things while you read this chapter:

- We are not trying to scare you with this information, and it is scary stuff to read.

- You can have your worries, your anxiety, your desire to not read this, *and* keep on reading.

The information here will help you detect the complications we discuss, prevent them from occurring, and treat those complications that can be treated.

Commit to your successful self-management by taking action!

Complication Prevention, Detection, and Treatment

One of the challenges with diabetes is that people are often diagnosed with the disease because a complication has already occurred. With most problems associated with diabetes, the real culprit is blood glucose levels being too high for too long. The problem is that no one really knows just how high is too high and for how long is too long. This is why everyone recommends that you be as consistent as you can in keeping your blood glucose levels in check and that your HbA$_{1C}$ levels remain as low as possible. These two things will help you prevent complications more than any one strategy alone.

The detection of many of these problems can actually be done fairly routinely by doctors trained to look for them. The best strategy you can employ here, besides keeping your blood sugars in good control, is to regularly see your specialist doctors who will examine you for the development of these problems. One of the rough things about having diabetes is that by the time *you* notice something doesn't seem right, a lot of damage has already been done. What you need is someone looking for the slightest evidence of these problems. Then, the issue of diabetes complications becomes much less complicated.

Some of the problems we will talk about here, even if they have developed already or end up affecting you, can be treated and even reversed. We are sure that you don't need us to say this, but it is generally better to prevent a problem than having to fix it once it does occur. Think about changing the oil in your car. As much of a nuisance and an expense as it can be, the whole purpose of changing the oil is really to prevent bad things from happening to your engine. Now, it may make your car "happier" or run better. It may be the "right thing to do," as a car dealer would tell us. But really, you change your oil to keep engine problems from developing. The time to realize you should change your oil needs to be before the engine seizes up on you, requiring a complete overhaul or brand-new engine. Still, there are replaceable parts for a car. Things can be restored.

This is true for some of the problems we address below. Just remember the oil example. A car almost never breaks down, seizes up, or otherwise stops working at a convenient time. Most people wish they had checked their oil, paid attention to the oil light coming and staying on, or had their car serviced regularly once bad things have already happened. Preventing and checking for complications and going to our version of a service shop (the doctor) will go a long way in keeping your diabetes uncomplicated.

Retinopathy: Looking Out for Your Eyes

Remember that retinopathy refers to problems with the retina of the eye, one of the most important parts of the eye and the part that lets you see. You know how important your eyes are. If you have experienced problems with your vision, you know this firsthand and better than we can describe it. Retinopathy can occur in a few versions. *Nonproliferative* or *background retinopathy* doesn't usually lead to vision loss, but left unchecked, it can lead to bigger problems. *Proliferative retinopathy* will lead to blindness if left untreated. As discussed in chapter 2, damage to the tiny blood vessels for the very small nerves in the eye can lead to permanent damage and vision loss.

Besides retinopathy, two other problems affect the vision of people with diabetes. These are more commonly talked about in our culture and are called *cataracts* and *glaucoma*. Now, you know that people without diabetes can have these problems as well. Unfortunately, people with diabetes are at a greater risk for getting them.

Cataracts affect our ability to see by partially (and sometimes completely) blocking light from entering the eye through the lens.

This clouding of the eye is not uncommon with the elderly, but people with diabetes can develop cataracts at an early age. With glaucoma, there is a problem of too much pressure inside the eye. This pressure can ultimately damage the very important pathway that carries information about what you see to your brain, called the *optic nerve*. Damage to the optic nerve can lead to permanent blindness. So, retinopathy, glaucoma, and cataracts can all lead to devastating consequences. That is definitely the bad news.

The good news is that all of these problems are detectable and largely treatable. With detection, the trick is to never let the problems get too far. Yearly eye exams are essential. This really needs to be a regular part of your diabetes management strategy. Your regular general practitioner is not going to be quite as skilled as an optometrist or ophthalmologist at detecting these types of eye problems, which makes sense, as optometrists and ophthalmologists are specially trained to examine your eyes.

In an eye exam, the optometrist or ophthalmologist will check for retinopathy, cataracts, and will do an intraocular pressure test for glaucoma. Each of these should be done yearly. Remember that prevention of these problems is essential. If you develop problems with your vision between visits, (pardon the pun here) get *seen* right away! In the event that a problem has developed, early detection and treatment is the best course. Eye problems will worsen with time, and detecting them in their earlier stages will make it less likely that you will experience permanent vision loss.

If problems have developed, there is still good news for your eyes. With cataracts, there is a fairly routine surgery to remove the cataract and affected lens and replace it with an artificial lens. With glaucoma, if detected early, the doctor can prescribe eyedrops that will help control the problem and likely prevent further vision loss. In the case of retinopathy, the story is not quite as optimistic. There are no drugs known to reverse the damage done from retinopathy. There are laser surgeries that can be used for this problem that will often result in some permanent vision loss, though not as bad as the retinopathy alone produces. Decreases in the amount you see (the field) and in night vision are also common with this type of surgery.

Nephropathy: Holding On to Your Kidneys

Your kidneys are a fundamental pair of organs. When you metabolize food and water your kidneys help rid your body of harmful by-products that occur as a result of this normal process. Your kidneys are essential for normal functioning. Initial damage to kidneys caused by diabetes can be detected by the increase in frequency and amount of urine you produce. This is because the kidneys are enlarged. While it may seem like they are working extremely efficiently judging by the amount you are urinating, you do not want them enlarged for long. This will cause damage and destruction to essential kidney cells.

An early detection test for kidney damage is called *clearance*. That is a pretty straightforward test for something called *hyperfiltration*, a rather more confusing sounding situation. However, the name is really just a technical way of talking about your kidneys working overtime for the reasons we just described; that is, they are doing their job of filtering (that's the "filtration" part of the word) but way too much (that's the "hyper" part). In this situation, the kidneys are swelling. Clearance is an easily done test (by your doctor, of course) to show if you are experiencing hyperfiltration. If this condition is present, you can likely reverse it by controlling and lowering your blood sugars. By doing this, more than half of the people diagnosed with hyperfiltration will avoid later stages of kidney disease. If you haven't already done so, you should schedule a clearance test with your doctor as soon as you can.

One of the ways to detect the next stage of kidney disease, or diabetic nephropathy, is with a urine test looking for *albumin*. Albumin, or protein in your blood, can show up in the urine in larger than normal amounts in the earliest stages of kidney disease. Unfortunately, there are no real signs or symptoms for you to notice that your kidneys are leaking blood protein into your urine. This is not something you can watch for on your own. As weird or terrifying as protein in the urine can sound, your doctor can very easily test for *microalbuminuria* (the fancy name for this condition). In fact, you should have a doctor screen you for this on a regular basis. Because the amount of protein we're talking about is so very small, even though it is more than normal, you may have a special screen for this requested by your doctor that requires several samples of urine. By doing a microalbuminuria test, you may be able to detect kidney disease several years before a regular urine dipstick could show that it is occurring.

Although this sounds unpleasant, the good news is that urine samples are one of the most painless procedures you can have done to detect one of the major problems you could face, namely, kidney damage. Be sure to tell your doctor if you have a history of urinary tract infections, as they can lead to damage as well. A microalbuminuria test should be done as soon as you are diagnosed with diabetes and once every year after that. If you haven't had this test done, go and do it now. We are serious. Get it checked now. *It's that important.* Left unchecked, this small amount of protein may lead to larger amounts of protein being leaked, and that is the beginning of real kidney disease. This will progress into kidney (also called *renal*) insufficiency and ultimately failure.

By testing for hyperfiltration, microalbuminuria, and the onset of kidney problems regularly, you may slow the process of kidney disease significantly. And here is some more good news: if you are able to prevent damage to your kidneys, the odds are very much in your favor that you will not develop retinopathy, or damage to your vision. The risks for both of these problems are lessened considerably by good glucose management.

Neuropathy: Where the Goal Is to Have a Lot of Nerve

In many ways, the story is similar for nerve damage complications due to diabetes. As described in chapter 2, neuropathy is the name given to nerve damage. You will more often hear the term (if anyone is talking about nerve damage, that is) *peripheral neuropathy*, referring to the peripheral nervous system. The peripheral nervous system sends information from the extremities (like hands and fingers and toes and feet) to the brain and also sends information from the brain to these areas. Let's take a moment to realize just how much we take our hands and feet for granted. If you place your hand near a hot surface, you should know about it right away. If you step on a tack (ouch!), you know immediately to get off of that tack and watch where you step next time.

Now, imagine if you didn't know you stepped on a tack because you had damage to the nerves in your foot. Believe it or not, you may not even notice you have a tack there. Then, you will likely not notice if you get an infection. (Face it—how often do we really look at the bottoms of our feet?) Diabetes puts people at higher risk for infection. This, coupled with poor circulation, means that a sore spot on the foot can get worse. And an infection could spread and ultimately lead to amputation, the surgical removal of the foot.

Alright, we are way ahead of ourselves. Amputation is certainly one of the worst-case scenarios. We need to concentrate on preventing and detecting these complications. You can dramatically reduce your chances of developing peripheral neuropathy by doing what you already know to do, namely, balance your diet, continue to exercise, and keep your blood sugars in control. Signs of peripheral neuropathy can include tingling (some call this "pins and needles") and numbness (loss of feeling) in your hands or feet. You may no longer be able to easily detect temperature. Some people report feelings of pain or even burning sensations in their skin. Your feet may swell, and you may experience cold hands and feet as symptoms of peripheral nerve damage. In more complex cases, some people notice problems with balance and an inability to know where their hands and feet are positioned relative to their body. Getting back to our foot example, some people will notice open sores or calluses on their feet. This can happen with your hands as well.

You can detect symptoms of nerve damage like these when they occur. However, your doctor or health care provider can test your reflexes and check your feet for you by testing them for sensitivity to temperature, touch, and vibrations. These tests may detect problems that are too slight for you to notice. They may also help remind you to really keep track of the sensitivity of your hands and feet.

The key, of course, is preventing this type of damage. What can you do? Well, aside from keeping your blood sugars in control, prevention requires taking good care of your body. This means not subjecting your hands and feet, in particular, to lots of stress. With your feet, you need to check them regularly for sores, blisters, and other wounds that are slow to heal or aren't clearing up. If you have trouble checking your feet, you can ask someone to help you with this. Another excellent idea is to make sure that you buy shoes that fit properly. Think about our car example from above. How long do you expect to be driving if you are not using reasonable tires, ones that fit and have good tread? Not long, right? Same goes for your feet, but with shoes. Also, avoid hot pavement and really cold temperatures on your feet. These can cause damage to your skin and result in the problems we just talked about. And make sure that your socks aren't too tight on your ankles, as this can cut down circulation to your feet. You really want to make sure you keep the blood flowing down there.

Another general rule about preventing neuropathy is to avoid drinking alcohol. Alcohol can damage your nerves, and with diabetes, that puts you at higher risk for problems. Alcohol not only disrupts your sense of balance, but the damage done to your nerves with diabetes and alcohol can cause permanent balance problems.

There are no known cures for peripheral neuropathy. There are medications that can help alleviate the pain and discomfort, but they will not reverse the damage. This is why detection and prevention (even of further problems) is so important. Types of medication that are prescribed often focus on alleviating the pain associated with neuropathy. These can include over-the-counter medications and those prescribed by your doctor. Some newer medications have been developed to specifically target pain associated with diabetes, and if this affects you, you may want to talk to your doctor about these options.

Additional strategies used by people with diabetes nerve pain include using a body stocking, pantyhose, or specially designed socks to prevent fabric and sheets from irritating and otherwise rubbing skin that has become more sensitive. Another excellent strategy to help alleviate nerve pain is one you already know to do—exercise! Walking, stretching, and even basic relaxation methods are very good ways to behaviorally reduce nerve pain. The good news is, if you are outside walking, not only are you helping with any nerve pain, but you are helping with your diabetes in general.

Cardiovascular Disease: Having a Heart, Circulation, and Everything Else!

Heart disease is a killer. While there are fewer deaths due to heart disease than there were in the past several decades, it's still a real problem (Fox et al. 2004). Unfortunately, it is an even bigger problem for people with diabetes. In fact, the risk of heart disease is twice that of people without diabetes and is even greater for women with diabetes than men with the disease (Bird et al. 2003; Lee et al. 2000). As you may know, the problem with heart disease is that it can lead to heart attacks. The problem with heart attacks is that they tend to kill people with diabetes even more than people without the disease. Keep reading, though, because there are things you can do to help keep this from happening.

Coronary Artery Disease

Coronary artery disease refers to the gradual closure of the arteries supplying blood to your heart. If these close completely, you will have a heart attack. Smoking, high blood pressure, and high cholesterol all interact to create coronary artery disease. These factors are an even bigger problem for people with diabetes. Detecting this type of heart disease can often occur by feeling a pain (called *angina*) or pressure in the chest during exercise or strenuous work. This is because the heart is using more blood. This pain can move around to the jaw or neck and even the left arm, shoulder, or armpit. Although the pain can happen if you exercise, it can also occur just sitting, waking up from sleep, and from emotional stress. Sometimes, though, coronary artery disease presents as abdominal discomfort and back pain. It can even feel like intense heartburn. If you have these symptoms, be certain to contact your doctor right away to discuss them.

Your doctor or health care provider may request a series of tests to help detect the presence of coronary artery disease. These can include an *electrocardiogram* (ECG) or an *echocardiogram* (also called a heart ultrasound). These tests can help detect the presence of coronary disease. It is really important, if possible, that you catch the disease in its earlier states. As it progresses unchecked, it can ultimately result in heart attack and death.

Strategies to treat heart complications can include oral medications such as nitroglycerin and beta-blockers. These drugs are designed to reduce symptoms and help prevent heart attacks. *Angioplasty* is another treatment given for coronary artery disease. This is a procedure done to help increase the size of openings in the arteries. Lastly, coronary artery bypass surgery may be performed to relieve angina and help improve the function of the heart. While there are potential complications with this surgical procedure (including postoperative infection), most people with diabetes do well with it.

Peripheral Vascular Disease

Other than to your heart, your arteries are supplying blood to many, many important parts of the body. When these arteries are clogged or damaged, it is referred to as *peripheral vascular disease.* Symptoms of peripheral vascular disease can include bodily pain such as in the calves, ulcers on the skin, and problems healing (particularly on the feet). Circulation to your extremities is fundamental to their survival. When circulation is lessened, problems result. If there is real artery blockage to your feet, your physician may discuss cleaning out the arteries surgically. Although this sounds dreadful, it is a very successful procedure for many people.

As we have already said in this chapter, the key is prevention. Preventing artery disease, be it of the heart or the hands or feet, begins with your physical health. Eating a balanced diet, reducing foods rich in cholesterol and fat, and increasing exercise are the primary keys to preventing most artery disease. If you have already been diagnosed with coronary artery disease, or even if you have had a heart attack, many of these problems can be stopped in their tracks by committing to and acting on a healthy lifestyle.

Sexual Dysfunction: Retaining Intimate Connections

You knew this section was coming. It's personal. It's hard to talk about. It's awkward for many of us. Still, sexual functioning is an essential part of human behavior, and *dysfunction* (when things go wrong) is cause for a great deal of concern. Unfortunately, with diabetes, sexual dysfunction is very common. We will talk first about the men, as they are much more frequently impacted by these problems. Then we'll address problems that women face in this area and issues related to sexual intimacy in a couple.

Sexual Dysfunction in Men

With men, the primary sexual problem that occurs in diabetes is *erectile dysfunction*; that is, difficulties obtaining and maintaining an erection. Although it can probably go unstated, problems with erections are determined by many, many factors. In theory, there are purely biological causes and purely psychological causes. However, these two factors interact so intricately that it's often very difficult to tease them apart. Said another way, it is possible to have problems with just the physical aspects of an erection, such as decreased circulation to the penis. However, worrying about getting an erection can contribute to difficulties obtaining and maintaining one. In either case, once a lack of erection when it was desired has occurred, many men get worried enough that it becomes increasingly unlikely one will happen.

With diabetes, circulation can be a problem. This makes it less likely that the physical mechanisms of having an erection are in good working order. Unfortunately, this problem increases the longer the man has diabetes, particularly if blood glucose is not well controlled. In addition, nerve damage (as discussed above) can decrease sensation in the penis, making it less likely an erection will occur. Certain heart medications, particularly those helping with blood pressure, can also decrease the likelihood of having an erection. In addition, medications prescribed for psychological difficulties such as depression have a very high likelihood of interfering with male sexual functioning.

There are several strategies that can be attempted to assist with this problem. The first issue concerns no longer drinking alcohol. Alcohol use can impair any man's ability to have an erection. Staying away from alcohol is a good part of healthy living and successful self-management of diabetes, and it may help with erectile dysfunction. There are medications that are prescribed for assisting with the erection process (physical stimulation is still required), but these can have dangers for people taking medications for heart problems. If you are interested in using these types of erection medications, be sure your doctor understands that you have diabetes and knows the interactions possible with the medications you take.

There are also numerous physical devices that have been developed to help men in this process. While this can be an uncomfortable thing to discuss, keep in mind that it is an incredibly well-researched area of medicine because it affects so many men. There are numerous options to discuss with your doctor, and one of them may be the perfect one for you.

Women and Sexual Dysfunction

For women with diabetes, sexual dysfunction is not as visibly noticeable as a man's erectile dysfunction. Still, women's sexual problems can be equally devastating and confusing. Problems women face in this area can include frequent yeast infections, which make sex painful or impossible. Although yeast infections are very treatable, getting more of them can also make a woman feel less sexual or intimate.

In addition, problems with circulation can cause a decrease in vaginal lubrication, as can peripheral neuropathy or nerve damage. When lubrication is decreased, the vagina may be less sensitive to touch and may be less responsive to sexual stimulation. In addition, for some women, lubrication is a psychological confirmation of engagement in the process; without this, a woman may feel less intimate, less connected, and less sexual in that moment. Aside from these basic reasons for its importance, decreases in vaginal lubrication can make sex painful.

Lastly, loss of skin sensation around the vagina due to peripheral neuropathy can reduce the experience of sexual pleasure. Like with men's sexual dysfunction, these problems are serious medical complications and, even if it's uncomfortable, should be discussed openly with your doctor. Unlike men's sexual dysfunction, however, there are fewer treatment options available for women at this time, so early detection and prevention are key.

The Psychology of Sexual Health

As we mentioned, sexual dysfunction is a complex process and is rarely solved with a single intervention. The psychological and social aspects of sexual relating are intricate, and we would not assume to be able to address all of those that could relate to any one individual or couple. There are numerous psychological issues that come to bear on sexual intimacy, including issues of trust, caring, and acceptance.

Some people with diabetes feel less attractive and less sexually desirable. These are very hard feelings to communicate for many people, and they may inhibit the sexual behaviors that might contribute to physical intimacy in a couple.

In addition, most people are raised to think of sex as performing or achieving (these terms are even part of some sex therapies!), and when a person does not "perform" the way he or she expects, disappointment follows. What's worse, many people are not sure what would please their partner or themselves.

Many people are too embarrassed or ashamed to talk about these issues. In fact, most of us are directly instructed that it's not appropriate to talk about sex by parents, family, friends, or whomever. Still, talking about these issues openly and honestly with all of the vulnerability you have will make a big difference in your partnership and your own sexuality.

Diabetes does not have to mean that sexual intimacy comes to a halt. There are many books right at your local bookstore that discuss thoughtful approaches to connecting in intimacy where sexual intercourse is actually no longer demanded or required in the process. Sensate focus is one such approach that concentrates on connection, relaxation, and gentle touching as a way to express love and affection. If these strategies don't work as well for you, consider talking to a counselor or psychotherapist as a couple. They often have many recommendations that will be much more specific to your situation. Sometimes couples therapy that focuses on very basic communication and conflict resolution can allow a couple to reconnect in sexual intimacy.

As we mentioned in chapter 2, psychological problems such as depression can have a profound impact on sexual functioning. In fact, for some people, lowered interest or desire for sex is simply a part of clinical depression. We end this chapter with a discussion of this common psychological issue.

Depression: Feeling Sad, Feeling Glad, Feeling What Is to Be Felt

Feeling bummed out, blue, melancholy, and generally sad about having diabetes is perfectly understandable. In fact, researchers suggest that feelings of depression are among the most common psychological problems experienced by people with diabetes (Rubin and Peyrot 1992). As described in chapter 2, feeling sad or depressed is a different phenomenon than what is called *clinical depression* or *major depressive disorder*. Clinical depression is a diagnosis that is characterized by having more than half of the nine main depression symptoms, that occur for at least two weeks, where you really don't have a day that goes by where you don't feel many of those symptoms. These symptoms include:

1. Having a depressed mood most of the day, nearly every day

2. Having less interest or pleasure in all, or almost all, activities that you used to enjoy most of the day, nearly every day

3. Having a significant change in weight (which can be either loss when not dieting or weight gain)

4. Having sleep problems like insomnia or sleeping excessively nearly every day

5. Being really slowed in your ability to move around or feeling like your behavior is agitated or restless

6. Feeling fatigued or having a loss of energy nearly every day

7. Feeling worthless or excessively (or inappropriately) guilty nearly every day

8. Having less ability to think or concentrate, feeling indecisive

9. Having recurrent thoughts of death, thoughts about committing suicide, attempting suicide, or having a specific plan for committing suicide

It's quite a list, and you may recognize thoughts or feelings you have had in that list. Depression really looks different in everyone. Some people experience many of the more "biological" looking symptoms like sleep problems and issues with weight, while others have more of the "psychological" symptoms such as sadness, guilt, and having problems concentrating. The bottom line is that depression is a hard set of feelings to experience.

What can make detecting depression challenging for people with diabetes is that the symptoms of diabetes can actually look a bit like the presentation of clinical depression. For example, confusion and fatigue can be a symptom of having your blood sugars out of control, and it is also a symptom of depression. One key difference is that with problems we would diagnose as depression, the difficulties are around most of the day, nearly every day, and other symptoms, such as sadness or depressed mood are also present. If you are not sure about this, you can talk to your health care provider. Make sure you tell them you are trying to separate out what is your diabetes from feeling clinically depressed.

The prevention of depression is a very complicated issue. Why is it that some people can survive really difficult problems and seem to bounce back while others sink into what looks like despair? Unfortunately, no one really knows. The experts aren't sure why some people get hit with major depressive disorder and some people don't.

Given that depression is relatively common among people with diabetes, perhaps there are a few suggestions to be made about staving off the blues. These suggestions work not only for preventing depression, but they are also tools used in clinical interventions.

Coping with Sadness and Depression

It is understandable if you find that you do not want to feel sad. Sadness is a very hard emotion for many of us to experience. What's more, we are often told to not feel sad, to stop crying, and to look on the bright side of things when we are around other people. One of the things you probably have noticed by now after reading this far is that sadness, or depression, is just a feeling, just like distress about diabetes. It's a feeling like any other that you wish wouldn't occur, but here it is. The question is: what do you want to do with this sadness? Maybe before you read this far, your answer was: "Do anything to make it go away." Hopefully, by this point, your answer at least includes bringing this sadness with you as you move in the direction of your values.

So if we take depression seriously, you may ask, how is it that we recommend not making it go away? The reason is partly related to the fact that depression is one of the most researched psychological problems that exists. This makes sense, given that it is very common and that it can be so debilitating for some people. One of the leading treatments out there is called behavioral activation, a component of many contemporary psychotherapies, which has been shown to be effective in reducing depression (Jacobson, Martell, and Dimidjian 2001; Lewinsohn et al. 1986; Martell, Addis, and Jacobson 2001). This means getting your body moving and engaging in activities that are meaningful and pleasurable for you. It turns out that just taking a walk and getting exercise can help people cope effectively with their sadness. Getting moving is not only consistent with how you are approaching your management of diabetes; it is a central part of your success!

Part of what works about getting active is that you frankly just feel better getting moving and spending time outside of the house (or work, or wherever). Another part of what makes behavioral activation so successful is that you get more chances to interact with other people. Now, many people who are depressed say the same thing to this last fact about social interactions. It sounds something like this: "But I don't want to interact with other people. Other people are why I am so depressed." It may be true that some of the people in your life are hard to interact with and those interactions may be part of your sad feelings, but not everyone is like that. In fact, just having an okay interaction with a stranger can help some people feel better. Our goal here is not to have you feel less sad or not sad at all. In fact, we want you to feel whatever you feel. What we want to suggest, though, is for you to get out and visit with the world. With your sad feelings. Take them with you. You may find that your feelings naturally move around, and you may even end up having a good day. In either case, you will be getting a little exercise in, and hey, that's part of your commitment for a healthy life.

We would really be remiss if we didn't remind you about what you read in chapter 9, Talking Diabetes. Although this isn't necessarily true for everyone in the world, most of us feel better talking about our struggles than keeping them inside. And, as you know, there are some real struggles with successfully managing your diabetes. Talking to others can be hard, but the payoff is often really large. As we have discussed before, sometimes other people are just waiting to help out, and sometimes they didn't even know you were upset and could really use a friend.

Getting More Help

If you think you could use some additional help with clinical depression, there are several options available to you. The leading two professional treatments are psychotherapy and medications. Both of these approaches are clinically proven to help most people with depression. Your chances of leaving depression behind after treatment, though, are greatly improved by having psychotherapy in combination with medications, or having just psychotherapy alone. Research now suggests that many people who just take medication may relapse back into depression when they stop taking it (Hollon et al. 2005).

Summing It Up

There are many complications associated with diabetes that can be very overwhelming to think about.

Many of these complications are treatable and preventable, but treatment and prevention require being educated and paying attention to symptoms.

The tools laid out in this book are designed to help you be able to pay attention to signs of complications, even if you are afraid, so that you can treat and prevent problems.

PART IV

Tying It All Together: Acceptance + Plan = Commitment

Chapter 12

Behavior Change

Throughout this book, we have tried to lay out a foundation for a way to have difficult thoughts, feelings, worries, concerns, nonmotivation, and anxiety and still take care of your diabetes if that is what you value. We have tried to also provide enough of the information you need to be able to live your values. For instance, if you value taking care of your diabetes by exercising, watching your diet, taking medications, and getting adequate support from people in your life to do so, we have tried to give you enough of the basic information to get started in a way that is best for you and your diabetes.

In this chapter and the next, we will attempt to integrate these two areas by helping you translate your values into an individualized plan that incorporates the latest information on the best ways to care for your diabetes and the tools you will need when you don't feel like taking care of it.

Choice

A key aspect of what we are asking you to do in this book is to live your life as a matter of choice, rather than because of reasons. This distinction may not make sense initially, so we'll try to explain what we mean by choice and reasons.

Reasons

When it comes to diabetes care, most people make all of their decisions based on the reasons they have in their head. These reasons can be positive or negative: "I take care of my diabetes because it makes me feel good about myself," or "I can't take care of my diabetes because I have no energy left after my busy day." These reasons often make a lot of sense and are very good reasons as far as reasons go.

Reasons as Causes

So if reasons are what we think about in terms of what enables our ability to do things or not, where does choice come in? *Choice*, for our purposes, is the direction you move in no matter what the reasons. For example, for the person who tells us that he takes care of his diabetes because it makes him feel good about himself, that person could still *choose* to not take care of his diabetes. And the person who tells us that she cannot exercise because she does not have the energy at the end of the day could still *choose* to go out and exercise, even if she didn't have the energy. This is what we mean by choice: moving in a direction regardless of the many reasons why you should or shouldn't move in that direction.

So what determines your choices, if not these reasons? That is the key question. The answer, of course, is your values.

If you think about it, we do this kind of choosing all the time in areas that aren't related to diabetes. Within marriages or committed relationships, we often choose not to have a romantic encounter with somebody else, even if we are tempted to, because we are choosing in the direction of our commitment. We may go to college, or take a difficult job, even if the extra work and stress are good reasons not to do it, because it has a higher meaning in relation to what we value for our lives and our achievements.

So why then would we talk about this so strangely, saying that we can make choices with or without reasons? Because reasons are very compelling. We often feel as though we are making choices completely because of the reasons that are there. We conceptualize life in the way it makes the most sense: that this causes that. In the examples above, we understand our not cheating on our partner due to the *reasons* that there would be consequences on the relationship or we would get caught. We understand our going to college or taking a difficult job as being *caused by* the practical need to make more money or achieve a certain level.

Undoing Cause-and-Effect Thinking

Given the compelling nature of reasons, it is especially important that we disconnect them from your ability to choose an action. If they remain stuck together, then as soon as the reasons change, the movement in the direction of your values could change. If you are only taking care of your diabetes because it makes you feel good about yourself, what happens if you wake up one day and it no longer makes you feel good about yourself? What if you find that you have developed a complication, despite your consistent work at it, and taking care of it now makes you feel bad instead of good? If the initial reason caused you to take care of yourself, then it would just be logical to now be in a situation where there was "no reason" to do it anymore. This might have especially negative consequences if the complication you developed could lead to more problems if you were not consistent with your self-care.

However, if you were taking care of your diabetes because doing so was consistent with your value to live a healthy life, it would matter less what your reasons were or if there were new reasons that seemed compelling. You would be able to continue to move forward toward your values.

Chessboard Revisited

One way to apply this to you and your own values is to think back to the Chessboard Exercise you first read about in chapter 5. Remember that we talked about the chessboard, which is you, as being able to do two things: to hold pieces and move in a direction. The pieces are all of the thoughts and feelings you have, whether positive or negative, and the direction of the board is determined by your values. You can choose to move the board in the general direction of your values, no matter what the "reasons" on the top of the board have to say. In fact, sometimes the negative thoughts and feelings ("I'll never be able to control my diabetes, so why even try?") might be winning the war taking place on the board, and sometimes the positive thoughts and feelings ("I can really keep my blood sugar down") are. This does not determine the course of the board at all, since the direction of the board is determined ahead of time by your goals and values.

Monsters on the Bus

An important metaphor within ACT treatment is that of the Monsters on the Bus (Hayes, Strosahl, and Wilson 1999). Many people find this helpful in making the distinction about choice and the role of reasons. Imagine that you are the driver of the bus that is your life. As the bus driver, you get to determine the route that you travel, and you carry around a number of passengers. Now, most of these passengers are friendly enough people, but there are a few in the back that are very scary. These passengers in the back look like monsters, and they have weapons and are dressed in scary black clothes that indicate that they mean business.

So imagine that as you're driving along on your route, you notice that they are starting to get a little restless in the back of the bus. And as you go along, they shout from the back that you should turn right at the light coming up. You had planned on going left, but you figure that if you go right, maybe they'll stay in the back of the bus and not mess with you. After a while, they again shout from the back that you should turn right. Worried that you will lose control of the route if you don't do something, you tell them that this time you will be turning left, not right. This agitates them even more, and they come up to the front of the bus so that you can't avoid them. They lean in and shout that if you don't turn right, something bad will happen. They look so scary and so real that you believe them, and you decide that it's not that big of a deal—so you turn right.

After a while, as you can imagine, all of the turns are right turns, and while the monsters haven't come back up to the front of the bus, you can't stop thinking about them. They are definitely determining your route. What you don't realize is that while they look very scary, they actually cannot hurt you, except in their capacity to make you feel things you don't want to feel and to have those feelings dictate your moving backward instead of forward in your life. As the driver, you are hoping for all of these monsters (or reasons) to change or get off the bus. Another solution that is hard to remember in the moment is that you can choose to turn left no matter what the monsters say, and while they might be difficult or scary, they cannot harm you.

Tony's Bus Ride

We saw a good example of how monsters can take over control of the bus with our patient Tony. Tony had struggled with his weight his whole life, and as a result he developed type 2 diabetes at the age of thirty-five. More than anything, Tony wanted to live his life healthfully and to enjoy every moment of life, something he thought was impossible to do until he had lost weight and gotten his health under control. When Tony found out that he had developed diabetes, he felt incredibly ashamed at his life being so out of control and so far from what he had dreamed of. He was embarrassed to tell anybody that he'd been diagnosed with diabetes, and he tried to just manage it on his own by throwing himself into a rigorous diet and exercise regimen. Not surprisingly, the enthusiasm for this difficult routine did not last long, and Tony soon added to his shame this most recent failed attempt to gain control of his health.

When Tony first came to see us, he had been turning "right" for so long, it took a while to define what he valued versus what he feared. Some days he'd say that he wanted to take care of his health, find a partner, and settle down and have a family. On other days he would say that he preferred to stay the way he was, and that he enjoyed having a life that was not full of the complexities of friendships and other important relationships. Ultimately, it became clear that even in meeting with us, the monster of "fear of trying again and failing" was attempting to steer the bus.

In order to really regain control of his bus and his health, Tony had to really feel that fear, as well as the embarrassment he felt about having diabetes and not being able to manage it through sheer force of will. When we talked about choice, Tony realized that one area where reasons (fear and embarrassment) were driving the bus was avoiding telling his friends and family about having diabetes. When we talked with him about what he would have to experience if he told them, he said that he would have to feel intense shame and embarrassment. When we asked him if he could choose to tell them even if he would have to feel these things, he said that he thought he could.

Not surprisingly, Tony's experience of telling his friends and family about his diabetes was nowhere near as bad as he had imagined it would be. He came in to our next meeting feeling buoyed by their support and ready to find other areas to turn "left" in his life. When we asked him about the embarrassment, he told us that it had been difficult and that the monsters had definitely been all the way up at the front of the bus trying to scare him. But he quickly realized that "nobody has ever actually died of embarrassment!"

Willingness as an Action

When we brought up the concept of willingness in chapter 6, we emphasized the role of willingness not as a feeling but as an action. The action of willingness is what making behavior change is all about: being willing with your feet to move forward in your life, even if it means discomfort or uncertainty. We say "with your feet" because, as we have talked about in previous chapters, sometimes you won't necessarily be willing with your head, and there will be plenty of reasons that you could come up with to be unwilling, but you can always still be willing with your feet.

Jumping

One of the best ways to describe what we mean by being willing with your feet to make changes in your life to better manage your diabetes is the idea of jumping (Hayes, Strosahl, and Wilson 1999). If you've ever had the experience of jumping off a diving board or a cliff into water, you probably know the sensation of being terribly unsure if this is a good idea—and then jumping anyway. As we get older, we tend to do a lot less "jumping," but we can usually remember what the sensation was like from when we jumped off things as a kid. Often, even though it is terrifying in the moments before you jump, there is something so exhilarating about the experience that it all seems worth it.

While your days of jumping out of trees or off cliffs may be over, we want to use the idea of jumping to help you think about making behavior changes to improve your life with diabetes. When you jump off something, there is no halfway; you can't half jump off a cliff or jump off the cliff with one foot still on the side. Also, when you jump off a high object, there is often plenty of fear there, but you can still jump with all that fear, and it may be worth the initial discomfort. Additionally, it doesn't matter how high off the ground the object is for the action to be the same; you can jump off a cliff or a building or a porch or a chair or a single piece of paper. The jumping motion is all the same. Finally, nobody can instruct you how to jump; it is something you learn by experience.

No Half-Willing

These properties of jumping make it a nice way to think about being willing with your feet. To start with, being willing isn't something that you can half do. If you aren't 100 percent willing (remember, this is "willing" as the behavior, not the feeling), then you are not willing. A good example of partial willingness was seen in a patient of ours named Sheila. She was a forty-two-year-old woman recently diagnosed with type 2 diabetes who came to us for help in making behavior changes to better manage her diabetes. Sheila definitely knew her stuff when it came to diabetes; she knew all of the carbohydrate counts for just about every type of food, she knew exactly how and how often to test her blood sugar, and, even though they were high, she kept a meticulous log of all of her values, and she knew exactly how exercise and weight lifting impacted her diabetes and knew when and how to take her medications. In short, she could have taught our diabetes patient–education classes for us.

So why was Sheila coming to see us? Because she would not jump. She always kept an emergency box of cookies in her cupboard and constantly kept part of herself from really making any of the behavior changes she knew were there for her to make. When we asked her about why that was, she said that she would be too vulnerable to failure if she let herself really start making those changes. She told us that if she always had a box of cookies on hand, she knew she always had a way to change her mind and it wasn't all so overwhelming. The problem was that since she always had an escape hatch, she was never really willing with her feet, and, as we mentioned, you can't jump with one foot still on the cliff.

Jumping with Fear

Another aspect of jumping that is reflected in being willing with your feet is the fact that even if you are unsure that you can accomplish your goals and ambitions, you can still be willing with your feet to move in their direction. Just as you can jump off the diving board with fear and terror, you can bring your fears and uncertainty with you as you move in a way that is willing. This idea was well-demonstrated by another patient, Chris, who was a thirty-eight-year-old man with diabetes who was referred to us because, despite developing the initial stages of circulatory problems related to his diabetes, he was unable to quit smoking. His smoking was directly impacting the development of his circulatory problems, and his doctors had told him for years that he was in danger of losing his feet (or worse) if he didn't stop smoking and improve his diabetes care. But Chris was unable to quit smoking no matter what he tried.

Part of the difficulty Chris had with quitting was the many rituals he'd developed that involved smoking. First, Chris would always stop at the local convenience store next to his work to buy his cigarettes in the morning. He had noticed that when he had tried to quit smoking, the urge to smoke a cigarette was overwhelming for him when he walked past the convenience store. He often gave up his attempts at that very spot because the craving was so strong.

In addition to this craving, Chris told us that his job was very stressful, and he would take several breaks a day to have a cigarette and relax. During the times that he had tried to quit he had realized that since he was not taking a break to have a cigarette, he was feeling much more stressed and exhausted at the end of the day. Thus, when he started to feel stressed during the workday, he would give up and go to the convenience store and (if he hadn't already done so when walking by that morning) buy a pack of cigarettes. Once he had bought a pack, he figured that he had blown it and he might as well smoke the rest of them.

Chris's story is a good example of how being willing with your feet requires some of the same actions as jumping off something high above the ground with lots of fear. In both instances, you have to be willing to tolerate an experience that you do not want to be having (fear or cravings) in order to do something you want to do. In Chris's case, he had to experience very strong cravings and discomfort. Rather than feel these things and still jump, he would climb down off the diving board and do what he could to reduce his discomfort. In short, he would move *away* from the cravings rather than *toward* his values.

Jumping Is Jumping

Another aspect of jumping that is similar to being willing with your feet is the fact that you can jump off any size object, and it is still jumping. The movement of jumping doesn't change whether you are jumping off a book or a cliff, and this element is also true of being willing with your feet. Often when patients come to see us, they have tried enormous feats in order to better manage their diabetes. They've eaten only 800 calories a day or run two hours every day until they inevitably failed, since maintaining that type of intensity is nearly impossible.

We often remind these and all our patients that being willing is the important muscle to build for long-term success, and that that muscle gets built by the practice of being willing over and over again. This means that smaller steps, like jumping off a book, are the best place to start for long-term achievement of your goals.

Jumping Is Not Verbal

Finally, the last aspect of jumping that is reflected in willingness is the fact that nobody can instruct you on how to jump. Imagine trying to explain to a child how to jump off of a step. You might be able to describe each of the movements involved: "first, bend your knees, but only about thirty degrees; then push off with the ball of your foot until your feet leave the step; then lift your feet up off the step, but then put them back down quickly again in order to have them under you for the landing." Even if you could describe every single step, the child probably wouldn't understand what you mean by "thirty degrees" or "ball of your foot" or many of the things in your instructions, and ultimately you would probably have to move their legs for them and abandon using language altogether.

Like this, we can try our best to describe what we mean by willingness here, but ultimately it is something that you must do to fully comprehend. Being willing with your feet is an experience, not a concept, and thus while we can try to describe what we mean by it, it is really only obtained by experiencing it.

Behavioral Momentum

One thing to remember when making difficult behavior changes is that the most effort is required in the beginning of the change. With just about any change of lifestyle, whether it's quitting smoking, exercising, eating right, or consistently testing your blood sugar, initiating the changes is typically much more difficult than maintaining them. When things disrupt the regular schedule, it becomes difficult again because the behavior must be reinitiated, but once you have a pattern of behavior going, you have what we call "behavioral momentum" (Nevin, Mandell, and Atak 1983).

What behavioral momentum literally means is that when you're starting a new behavior, after a certain number of times of doing it, you have created a habit. Once you have a habit, whether it's positive or negative, it becomes easier to do that thing regularly. Thus, while making behavior changes may feel difficult now, it's only a matter of time before you have behavioral momentum on your side and instead of having a habit of eating potato chips in front of the television, you get accustomed to taking a walk before dinner.

In order to capitalize on this behavioral momentum, of course, you have to start a new behavior or lifestyle change. As we have talked about throughout this book so far, this often brings with it many "reasons" or "pieces" or "passengers," from fear of failure to the thought that it will never get any better. And as we have covered in previous chapters, the most important weapon in overcoming these barriers is getting practice in taking new steps *with* all these thoughts and feelings.

To do that, we suggest that you revisit the Willingness Exercise you attempted (or considered) in chapter 6. That exercise asked you to think of one small step that you could take that would bring all of the uncomfortable thoughts and feelings up for you, so that you could practice responding differently to them and move in the direction of your values.

Were you able to accomplish the goal you set out for yourself? It's okay if you weren't, or if you meant to but didn't end up implementing the goal. That happens a fair amount even with patients who come in to see us in the office. If you did not attempt it, it's worth taking a look again at what barriers you encountered. If you did attempt it, how did it go? Did uncomfortable thoughts and feelings come up? If so, how did you handle them?

Regardless of whether you were able to reach the goal you set for yourself last time, it's time to continue to move forward in the direction of your values. In order to do this, we invite you to again spend some time thinking about what means the most to you in terms of your values in your relationships, what you spend your time doing, and your health.

If you were not able to achieve the goal you set for yourself in the last exercise, think about what is most meaningful in terms of your valued direction and come up with one small goal that you think you can achieve in order to move in that direction. This "turning left" may again bring up some monsters from the back of the bus, but with your increasing ability to just notice these thoughts and feelings and the mindfulness practice you have been using, the presence of these discomforts hopefully will not serve as barriers this time.

Willingness Exercise II

If you were able to accomplish the goal you set in the first willingness exercise, see if you can take it one step further: see if you can take a slightly higher jump this time. It's okay if you're not able to achieve it right away; remember, it should be a goal that requires you to feel or experience a thought, sensation, or urge that ordinarily would serve as a barrier to your attempting the action. Write down in your diabetes journal what you will be attempting.

Now write down what thoughts, feelings, or urges you will need to be willing to have in order to do this.

Summing It Up

Long-term behavior change involves choosing to move in a direction, no matter what the reasons are to do otherwise.

Being willing with your feet, even when you don't feel like keeping up behavior changes, requires many of the same elements as jumping off a high place.

CHAPTER 13

Stand and Commit

One thing patients often ask about is the name of this treatment approach: acceptance and commitment therapy. By the time we have reached the end of treatment when patients are meeting with us, they tell us that they now understand what we mean by acceptance; that the purpose of what we have been talking about so far is to accept thoughts and feelings, even the ones you don't really want to accept, so that you can move in a valued direction.

But the concept of commitment is often a trickier one. We had one patient who claimed at the beginning of the treatment group that he had joined because he had "commitment issues." He explained that since he had ended many relationships when they seemed to be getting serious, his doctor had recommended this group to him to help him accept these issues so that he could focus on his diabetes management.

While our patient (and his doctor) was probably just guessing at the purpose of the group based on popular definitions for the words in the name of the treatment, he had a point in one sense: he did have commitment issues, just like many of us do, and his doctor had recommended the group to help him address them. Of course we don't necessarily mean difficulty committing to long-term relationships when we say "commitment issues," the way this patient probably did. We mean that making and keeping commitments to lifestyle changes is very difficult for most people, and in that sense we all have issues with commitment.

The reason we use the word "commitment" when talking about behavior changes is that, as we all know, it is one thing to know that a behavior change needs to be made, and even to have the tools to be mindful of all of the negative thoughts and feelings that might get in the way of making that behavior change and making it anyway. It's a whole different ball game to then implement those changes in your life day in and day out. Making changes permanent requires something extra. That extra piece is what we talk about as *commitment*: committing to make changes regardless of what reasons appear.

A good example of how this pertains to diabetes-related behaviors can be seen with the case of Nancy, a fifty-three-year-old woman who was referred to us when she was first diagnosed with type 2 diabetes for help in making behavioral changes. After working with Nancy for only a couple of weeks, it was clear to us that she was a natural with this approach. She very quickly was able to notice her thoughts and feelings *as* thoughts and feelings, and she so clearly identified with each of her values that we thought we would not be seeing Nancy for long, since she wouldn't need our help for more than a few meetings to be on the path to good diabetes management.

After about a month, however, we started to notice a pattern with Nancy's diabetes care that concerned us. She had identified values and goals related to her health that included cutting back on sweets to only two servings per week, increasing the servings of green vegetables she ate per day from zero to two, and working up to a forty-five-minute walk each morning before going to work. After each meeting with us, she would do a great job of sticking to these goals for a day or two, but then her motivation would flag and by the time she came to see us again, she would have abandoned all of her efforts. Then, we would talk about what had worked and what hadn't and spend some time helping her make room for her thoughts that said if she didn't stick to her goals perfectly, then she might as well throw them out the window. If she could allow these thoughts to be on the bus with her, she would be able to slip up and still move in the direction of her values. But, try as we might, Nancy would leave and accomplish her goals for a few days, and then it would all start over again.

We soon realized that understanding the principles or defining her goals and values was not the problem for Nancy—making a commitment to these lifestyle changes was. She was making small changes for a couple of days, but only in order to be able to come back and tell us she had succeeded, not because she was committed to living a life that was meaningful and value driven for her. When she came into the next session with the same results, we were careful not to provide feedback one way or the other on her performance. We spent the entire meeting talking about what would be a meaningful life for her and having her write a story portraying a day in the most meaningful life imaginable for her. When she did, she quickly identified that she wanted to make a commitment to living that life that included less junk food, more healthy food, and more exercise, rather than to the idea of pleasing us or meeting arbitrary goals she had set for herself.

Nancy's case is a good example of how just making behavioral changes is not enough; the extra step that is needed at this point is to make a commitment to continuing to move in the direction of your values, even when things are hard or you get knocked off track.

Making a Commitment

The concept of making a commitment sounds good in theory, but what is actually involved? Below we have broken down the process of making a commitment into a number of steps. Not all of the steps will necessarily apply in every case. For instance, some people prefer to make commitments and behavior changes without the use of outside support or support groups, while for other people this is a crucial part of how they will make and maintain their commitments.

Saying What You Commit To

For our purposes here, the first step in making a commitment is defining your values and determining what direction they lead you in. Much of this first step has been the focus of this book and our efforts to help you define what you value. Often, we don't have any idea what is important to us until we go through this journey, and what exactly we think is important in terms of our behavior is often a topic we'd rather not explore for fear that we will find ourselves lacking.

Once your values have been defined, the second step is to make a commitment to move in their direction. This can be overwhelming, and often we find that patients would rather simply take their values into consideration when deciding how to behave rather than make a strong commitment to these values. One patient who had difficulty with this step was Alex, a forty-five-year-old man with type 2 diabetes who came to us for help in managing his out-of-control sugar levels. Like Nancy, Alex did not have a difficult time noticing his thoughts and feelings and was able to clearly define what was important to him in the values-clarification portion of our work with him. He had two small children and was very motivated to make behavioral changes to get to see them grow up, get married, and have children of their own.

When it came to making a commitment, however, Alex suddenly felt much more uncertain. When we explored what this hesitance was about, he told us that he realized that once he made a commitment to making behavior changes, that was it: he could no longer pretend that these things didn't matter to him, and he could no longer pretend that it was not a big deal if he ate an entire bag of cookies. He told us that making a commitment, and tying that commitment to his desire to be a part of his kids' lives for as long as possible, would make him feel terrible every time he had a slip, and he just didn't know if he was ready to make all of these changes all at once in his life.

His apprehension made a lot of sense to us. It would be very overwhelming to have all of the pressure of living a meaningful life be dependent on making certain changes. If he were unable to make those changes, or even had days where he slipped up, it would feel as though he were giving up the idea of living a meaningful life. We talk about understanding slipups below, but it's important to remember that we're not talking about committing to a specific outcome here; the point of committing is to commit to living a life that is headed in the direction of your values. This commitment is a way to help orient your behavior and bring wonderful things to your life, not to serve as a threat to hold over your head.

Doing What Works

Perhaps the best way to describe what we mean when we talk about committing is the idea of determining whether or not something is working for you in your life and making a commitment to move in the direction of things that are working. By "working" we mean whether or not they are moving you toward or away from living your values. In Alex's case, the behaviors that worked for him in his life in terms of his values were things like taking a walk when he wanted to eat an entire bag of cookies and managing his diabetes every day. Rather than asking him to commit to taking those specific actions, we were asking him whether he could make a commitment to have those values be the direction he was heading, whether he slipped up or not.

Talking About It

Another important step in making a commitment of any type is to talk about it. Talking about your commitment can mean a number of different things, and we cover two examples, telling people in your life and getting support, below. Essentially, talking about your commitment and your values is a way to let people help you continue to move in a direction that works for you. This can be especially important for people with diabetes, since the number of times per day decisions must be made regarding valued behaviors is so high. For instance, letting people know that you are committed to moving in a direction that is consistent with your value of good health and good diabetes care can give people the opportunity to support you in staying on track.

Telling People Who Are Important to You

Probably the most important people to talk with about your commitment are the people in your life. Whether it's friends, family, coworkers, or neighbors, letting the people around you know what is important to you and about your willingness to experience discomfort in order to live according to your values is often crucial to being able to sustain committed action.

Admittedly, however, telling people in your life about your commitment is often a complicated prospect. Telling friends and family may provide opportunities for support in making valued choices, but it also provides opportunities for criticism and evaluation, which many people prefer to avoid. Take the example of Rose, a forty-six-year-old woman diagnosed with type 2 diabetes who came to see us for help in making the lifestyle changes her doctor had recommended. Rose told us that while she felt ready to commit to making behavioral changes and to live her values *with* all of the "pieces," she had about not being able to do it, she didn't feel that she could make that commitment public to her friends and family. When we asked her why, she told us that she worried that they would evaluate everything she did and everything she ate, and that her private moments of "failure" would be made worse by having others see not only that she was doing things that were not good for her diabetes, but that she was doing so after publicly stating her commitment to move in the opposite direction.

Upon hearing this, we asked Rose what she thought was the most workable of the two choices she had—to talk with her friends and family or not talk to them. We reminded her to keep in mind that we were using "workable" to mean which one would help her live her values. She told us that the thing that seemed as though it would be most useful or workable in helping her live her values would be to tell everybody so that they could help her. She also felt that knowing that the people in her life knew what she was going for would help keep her on track so that she could avoid their evaluation. Then we asked her, given this, what the cost would be of telling them. She quickly identified that the cost would be that she would have to feel negative feelings, shame and embarrassment specifically, when she slipped. Before we could ask anymore questions, Rose then smiled and said that she was again at an intersection, with her values going in one direction and her desire to not ever have to feel negative feelings heading in the other. She told us that since she knew that choosing to tell her friends and family was the direction that would most help her live her values, she was willing to have all of the negative feelings that might come from their evaluation if it meant moving one step closer to living her values.

Finding and Getting Support

Another way to talk about your commitments is to find places to get support from other people struggling with the same issues. There are millions of people with diabetes in the United States alone, and there are countless online and community resources for people seeking a connection with others living with diabetes. A great resource for connecting with others with diabetes in the United States and internationally is the American Diabetes Association website at www .diabetes.org. More often than *how* to contact resources, however, our patients ask us *why* they should think about contacting one of these organizations. To answer that, we often first point out that everybody is different, and what is helpful for one person may not be helpful for another. Remember, the key here is whether or not something works to better help you live your values, and workability is typically defined individually.

However, we have noticed that finding ways to get support from other people with diabetes can be helpful in moving in a valued life direction for some. The principle for why this is the case is related to our discussion in chapter 9 about talking with friends and family about your diabetes. Other people living with diabetes not only understand your experiences and struggles and can empathize with your situation, but they also tend to be more skeptical about reasons as causes of behavior and are more likely to help you in your taking care of your diabetes even when it feels as though the barriers are insurmountable.

We have often heard from patients that while these groups might be helpful, they can also be stressful for some people, since there may be members with complications more severe than your own and having to be aware of these complications in person or online generates more fear and stress than the support from the community relieves. In addition, we have had patients who state that they really are not joiners, and that these groups are full of "diabetes freaks" and people whose whole lives are focused on their diabetes.

Again, while we have lots of room for individual variability in whether or not something works, we often point out to these patients that they are rejecting a potential source of support in moving toward their values because of wanting to avoid feelings or thoughts—thoughts about what type of person they are, about what type of people belong to the group, or thoughts about what will or will not be helpful. Instead of buying these thoughts as true simply because they are there, we encourage patients to go and see what their experience tells them. Often, they come back to say that they are grateful they checked with their experience because, once again, they discovered that they could have their worries while they moved forward in the direction of their values.

Choosing Each Day

Another key step to making and keeping a commitment is to choose each day to live in the direction of your values and commitments. This involves choosing to exercise even when the urge not to is really strong, because you are committed to moving in the direction of your values. It also means keeping in mind that you can continue to choose to move in a direction whether you slipped up the day before or not. Choosing, like being willing with your feet, is not necessarily something that you need to fully understand in order to do, but rather is something that you do each day. That is committing to living your values fully.

Relapse

Understanding slipups or relapses is an important part of making and keeping commitments in the long term. It's important to remember that while slipups will happen from time to time, what you are committing to is not necessarily a specific set of outcomes but rather the *process* of letting your values guide your behavior. There will be times when you head away from your fears or urges rather than in the direction of your values, but commitment is about noticing these times and redirecting yourself toward your values.

Commitment Exercise

In the introduction we told you that picking up this book was the first step toward moving from a life of existing to a life of really living. Making a commitment toward living a life directed by values, in diabetes care as well as the rest of your experiences, is what we meant by that. The final task in this process is to fully define and write down what that means for you in your life and to make the commitment to live those values. The way to do that is to spend some time thinking about what it means for you to live your most important values and to have meaning in your life, and then to make a written commitment to live those values in your life.

The reason that it's important to actually write down your commitments (preferably in your diabetes journal) is that this act of writing will allow you to firmly define what direction you want to commit to in your life, and it will provide you with a concrete resource to look back on later. Also, writing in this way can really help you to put your thoughts, fears, and commitments into words, which will assist in your own understanding and help in talking about your values and commitments with others.

The form your commitment takes may vary, but for most people, the written commitment starts with the sentence, "I am committed to living a life that is ..." and then describes the direction you want to move in your life. It also helps to mention how you'd like to manage your thoughts and feelings that come up, especially those that feel as though they could interfere with your living your life in this way. For instance, you may write that you are committing to taking care of your diabetes through exercise, diet, testing, and medication management in order to live a healthy and full life with diabetes, and you're committing to take care of your relationships by being a thoughtful, caring friend, partner, or family member. Further, you might state that you are committing to letting these values determine the direction you move, rather than your fear or worry, and that when these emotions occur, you are committed to working on noticing them rather than needing to eliminate them.

Now, take some time to consider what you would like to commit to. Then, when you have a good idea, write in your diabetes journal what direction you commit to move in, being as specific as possible about your values and what would be a meaningful life for you.

Then write down what you commit to do with difficult feelings or thoughts that show up as you move toward these values.

Moving Forward from Here

The information and skills talked about in this book are designed to help you live an amazing life with diabetes. We know that from here on out your life will include some ups and some downs, as all lives do. But we hope that the framework laid out in this book will give you the tools to experience difficult or uncomfortable feelings related to your diabetes and other areas of your life without having to avoid or eliminate them, allowing you to use your values as a guide for moving forward. Remember, each day you have everything it takes to live a meaningful life *with* your diabetes!

Summing It Up

Commitment involves stating to yourself and to others the values you hold and making a promise to move in that direction.

Difficult thoughts and feelings will come up and get in the way of moving in your committed direction, but the commitment to living an amazing life with diabetes is made to this process, not to any one outcome.

References

American Psychiatric Association. 2000. *Diagnostic and Statistical Manual of Mental Disorders*. 4th ed. Washington, DC: American Psychiatric Association.

Bird, C. E., A. Fremont, S. Wickstrom, A. S. Bierman, and E. McGlynn. 2003. Improving women's quality of care for cardiovascular disease and diabetes: The feasibility and desirability of stratified reporting of objective performance measures. *Women's Health Issues* 13:150-57.

Centers for Disease Control and Prevention. 2005. *National Diabetes Fact Sheet: General Information and National Estimates on Diabetes in the United States, 2005*. Atlanta, GA: Department of Health and Human Services, Centers for Disease Control and Prevention.

Clark, D. M., S. Ball, and D. Pape. 1991. An experimental investigation of thought suppression. *Behaviour Research and Therapy* 29:253-57.

Cowie, C. C., K. F. Rust, D. D. Byrd-Holt, M. S. Eberhardt, K. M. Flegal, M. M. Engelgau, S. H. Saydah, D. E. Williams, L.S. Geiss, and E. W. Gregg. 2006. Prevalence of diabetes and impaired fasting glucose in adults in the U.S. population: National Health and Nutrition Examination Survey 1999–2002. *Diabetes Care* 29:1263–68.

Diabetes Control and Complications Trial Research Group. 1993. The effect of intensive treatment of diabetes on the development and progression of long-term complications in insulin-dependent diabetes mellitus. *New England Journal of Medicine* 329:977-86.

Fox, C. S., S. Coady, P. D. Sorlie, D. Levy, J. B. Meigs, R. B. D'Agostino Sr., P. W. Wilson, and P. J. Savage. 2004. Trends in cardiovascular complications of diabetes. *Journal of the American Medical Association* 292:2495-99.

Gregg, J. A., G. M. Callaghan, S. C. Hayes, and J. L. Glenn-Lawson. Forthcoming. Improving diabetes self-management through acceptance, mindfulness, and values: A randomized controlled trial. *Journal of Consulting and Clinical Psychology.*

Hardy, R. R. 2000. *ZenMaster: Practical Zen by an American for Americans.* Tucson, AZ: Hats Off Books.

Hayes, S. C., and S. Smith. 2005. *Get Out of Your Mind and Into Your Life.* Oakland, CA: New Harbinger Publications.

Hayes, S. C., K. D. Strosahl, and K. G. Wilson. 1999. *Acceptance and Commitment Therapy: An Experiential Approach to Behavior Change.* New York: Guilford Press.

Hollon, S. D., R. J. DeRubeis, R. C. Shelton, J. D. Amsterdam, R. M. Salomon, J. P. O'Reardon, M. L. Lovett, P. R. Young, K. L. Haman, B. B. Freeman, and R. Gallop. 2005. Prevention of relapse following cognitive therapy vs. medications in moderate to severe depression. *Archives of General Psychiatry* 62:417-42.

Jacobson, N. S., C. R. Martell, and S. Dimidjian. 2001. Behavioral activation treatment for depression: Returning to contextual roots. *Clinical Psychology: Science and Practice* 8(3):255-70.

Jahromi, M. M., and G. S. Eisenbarth. 2006. Genetic determinants of type 1 diabetes across populations. *Annals of the New York Academy of Sciences* 1079:289-99.

Lee, W. L., A. M. Cheung, D. Cape, and B. Zinman. 2000. Impact of diabetes on coronary artery disease in women and men: A meta-analysis of prospective studies. *Diabetes Care* 23:962-68.

Lewinsohn, P. M., R. F. Muñoz, M. A. Youngren, and M. A. Zeiss. 1986. *Control Your Depression*. Englewood Cliffs, NJ: Prentice-Hall.

Lovejoy, J. C. 2002. The influence of dietary fat on insulin resistance. *Current Diabetes Reports* 2:435–40.

Martell, C. R., M. E. Addis, and N. S. Jacobson. 2001. *Depression in Context: Strategies for Guided Action*. New York: W. W. Norton.

Mason, N. J., A. J. Jenkins, J. D. Best, and K. G. Rowley. 2006. Exercise frequency and arterial compliance in non-diabetic and type 1 diabetic individuals. *European Journal of Cardiovascular Prevention and Rehabilitation* 13:598-603.

Nevin, J. A., C. Mandell, and J. R. Atak. 1983. The analysis of behavioral momentum. *Journal of the Experimental Analysis of Behavior* 39:49-59.

Pate, R. R., M. Pratt, S. N. Blair, W. L. Haskell, C. A. Macera, C. Bouchard, D. Buchner, W. Ettinger, G. W. Heath, and A. C. King. 1995. Physical activity and public health: A recommendation from the Centers for Disease Control and Prevention and the American College of Sports Medicine. *Journal of the American Medical Association* 273:402-7.

Rosamond, W., K. Flegal, G. Friday, K. Furie, A. Go, K. Greenlund, N. Haase, M. Ho, V. Howard, B. Kissela, S. Kittner, D. Lloyd-Jones, M. McDermott, J. Meigs, C. Moy, G. Nichol, C. J. O'Donnell, V. Roger, J. Rumsfeld, P. Sorlie, J. Steinberger, T. Thom, S. Wasserthiel-Smoller, and Y. Hong. 2007. Heart disease and stroke statistics—2007 update: A report from the American Heart Association Statistics Committee and Stroke Statistics Subcommittee. *Circulation* 115:e69-e171.

Rubin, R. R., and M. Peyrot. 1992. Psychosocial problems and interventions in diabetes: A review of the literature. *Diabetes Care* 15:1640-57.

Stern, L., N. Iqbal, P. Seshadri, K. L. Chicano, D. A. Daily, J. McGrory, M. Williams, E. J. Gracely, and F. F. Samaha. 2004. The effects of low-carbohydrate versus conventional weight loss diets in severely obese adults: One-year follow-up of a randomized trial. *Annals of Internal Medicine* 140:778-85.

Stewart, K. J. 2002. Exercise training and the cardiovascular consequences of type 2 diabetes and hypertension: Plausible mechanisms for improving cardiovascular health. *Journal of the American Medical Association* 288:1622-31.

Temelkova-Kurktschiev, T. S., C. Koehler, E. Henkel, W. Leonhardt, K. Fuecker, and M. Hanefeld. 2000. Postchallenge plasma glucose and glycemic spikes are more strongly associated with atherosclerosis than fasting glucose or HbA$_{1C}$ level. *Diabetes Care* 23:1830-34.

Tuomilehto, J., J. Lindstrom, J. G. Eriksson, T. T. Valle, H. Hamalainen, P. Ilanne-Parikka, S. Keinanen-Kiukaanniemi, M. Laakso, A. Louheranta, M. Rastas, V. Salminen, and M. Uusitupa. 2001. Finnish Diabetes Prevention Study Group: Prevention of type 2 diabetes mellitus by changes in lifestyle among participants with impaired glucose tolerance. *New England Journal of Medicine* 344:1343–50.

UK Prospective Diabetes Study Group. 1998. Intensive blood-glucose control with sulphonylureas or insulin compared with conventional treatment and risk of complications in patients with type 2 diabetes (UKPDS 33). *Lancet* 352:837-53.

Vitaliano, P. P., J. M. Scanlan, J. Zhang, M. V. Savage, I. B. Hirsch, and I. C. Siegler. 2002. A path model of chronic stress, the metabolic syndrome, and coronary heart disease. *Psychosomatic Medicine* 64:418–35.

Jennifer Gregg, Ph.D., is a clinical psychologist and assistant professor in the Department of Psychology at San Jose State University in San Jose, CA. She completed her Ph.D. at the University of Nevada, Reno, and did her pre- and postdoctoral training at the Veteran's Administration hospital in Palo Alto, CA. She has authored many articles and book chapters in the areas of chronic and terminal disease, applications of acceptance and commitment therapy, and the treatment of psychological disorders in primary care medical settings. In addition to teaching, supervision, and research activities, she has a private practice and provides training in acceptance and commitment therapy in the San Francisco Bay Area.

Glenn M. Callaghan, Ph.D., is professor of psychology at San Jose State University and a member of the Association for Behavioral and Cognitive Therapies and Western Psychological Association. He is an expert in functional analytic psychotherapy and functional assessment methodology. He has published multiple articles in the areas of psychotherapy process and alternative approaches to assessment of psychological distress.

Steven C. Hayes, Ph.D., is University of Nevada Foundation Professor of Psychology at the University of Nevada, Reno. He has authored more than 350 articles and book chapters and numerous books, including *Get Out of Your Mind and Into Your Life, Acceptance and Commitment Therapy,* and *Relational Frame Theory.* A past president of the Association for Behavioral and Cognitive Therapies, he has conducted hundreds of trainings in ACT around the world and supervised the training of hundreds of graduate students.

Foreword writer **Michael Singer, MD,** is a perinatal obstetrician and consultant gynecologist with East Bay Perinatal Medical Associates and Alta Bates Medical Center, both in Berkeley, CA

more titles for **living a more healthful lifestyle**
from new**harbinger**publications

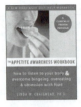
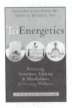
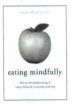
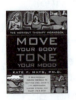
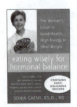